HEALING CANCER

HEALING CANCER

Complementary Vitamin & Drug Treatments

DR ABRAM HOFFER, MD, FRCP(C)
WITH LINUS PAULING, PHD

CCNM PRESS

The publisher acknowledges the support of the Government of Canada, Department of Canadian Heritage, Book Publishing Industry Development Program.

The publisher does not advocate the use of any particular treatment program, but believes that the information presented in this book should be available to the pubic. The nutritional, medical, and health information presented in this book is based on the research, training, and personal experiences of the author, and is true and complete to the best of the author's knowledge. However, this book is intended only as an informative guide to those wishing to know more about good health. It is not intended to replace or countermand the advice given by the reader's physician. Because there is always some risk involved, the author and the publisher are not responsible for any adverse effects or consequences from any of the suggestions made in this book. And because each person and each situation is unique, the author and the publisher urge the reader to consult with a qualified professional before using any procedure where there is a question as to its appropriateness.

ISBN 1-897025-11-4

Edited by Bob Hilderley.
Design by Sari Naworynski.

Printed and bound in Canada.

Published by CCNM Press Inc., 1255 Sheppard Avenue East,
Toronto, Ontario M2K 1E2 Canada.
ccnmpress@ccnm.edu

CONTENTS

ACKNOWLEDGEMENTS

To Bob Hilderley for his very skillful editing of a very complicated manuscript. This is my fourth book edited by Bob, and each time I am more impressed with his editorial skill. It is becoming easier and easier for me and I am sure more and more difficult for Bob, but he succeeded in making this book much more legible and much more interesting, while retaining the scientific accuracy of what Dr Linus Pauling and I wrote.

I also dedicate this book to Linus Pauling, the greatest modern scientist, for his immense contribution to the theory and practice of orthomolecular psychiatry and medicine, and for his steadfastness and determination not to be diverted by the "hordes" of critics. The father of modern bedside medicine, Sir T. Sydenham, once wrote, "A medical discovery is like a sapling in the middle of the King's highway. If it is not fenced in, it will be trampled by the galloping hordes." He was asking for help from one of the nobility about 300 years ago because he had discovered that small pox was best treated by decreasing the fever, not by increasing it, as had been the custom for the previous 1,500 years.

Linus Pauling was such a medical discoverer. If I had the power, I would have given him an Honorary MD, to add to his dozens of Ph.D.s and DScs.

I also must acknowledge the help and education I received from more than 1,000 patients with cancer I have seen over the past 23 years, especially to Miss A.S., Case Number 84, born in 1919, first seen for her pancreatic cancer in July 1978, who died 19 February, 1999. She turned my professional career around.

Finally, I acknowledge the help given to me by Fran Fuller, who has for the past 22 years carefully and methodically kept my charts and maintained the records so that it is possible to keep the database in my computer up-to-date with minimum effort.

Thanks to you all, friends and colleagues.

Abram Hoffer

PREFACE

Several years ago I attended a festschrift celebrating the life and career of Dr Arthur Sackler where I met my old friend and colleague Linus Pauling in his hotel room, next to mine. He had just finished breakfast with his son Linus Jr, and I found him with a hand calculator doing some calculations. He told me he was recalculating electron orbitals, adding that he was able to understand them better by doing his own calculations. During our conversation, I told him that I had discovered that he and Dr Ewan Cameron were correct in their claim in their book *Cancer and Vitamin C* that vitamin C in optimum dosage was effective for the treatment of cancer. During the previous decade I had prescribed megadoses of vitamin C and other nutrients for patients suffering from various forms of cancer and the results showed this treatment to be very effective, not only in extending the lives of patients but also in improving the quality of their lives. Dr Pauling asked me whether I intended to publish my findings, but I replied that I did not, noting that given the adverse response from the established medical community to his reports on the efficacy of megavitamin treatment, there was no point in preparing a report since no medical journal would accept it for publication. Nevertheless, he urged me to proceed with more careful studies on the much larger group of patients and promised to help me find a journal that would publish. I agreed to this plan, but when I arrived home, I changed my mind, for I did not relish the massive work involved in doing a large scale follow-up study and I was not certain Dr Pauling was serious, thinking that perhaps he was simply being kind to an old friend. Two years later, I received a letter from Linus asking me for the data I had agreed to prepare. I promptly apologized and completed a follow-up study on the first 134 patients I had seen over a 10-year period since 1978.

In the meantime Dr Pauling had become interested in methods of calculating probable outcome using cohorts of patients based upon the Hardin Jones biostatistical method. He applied this method to the data I had sent him. My examination of the data convinced me that the patients on a megavitamin regimen had a much better outlook. His examination was much more detailed and showed a very significant improvement of the treated compared to the untreated group. We published the results of this and a subsequent study in the *Journal of Orthomolecular Medicine.* Later we co-authored a further report published in the same journal.

After Linus Pauling and I published our first account of cancer patients treated with high dose vitamin C and other nutrients, we planned to write a book detailing our results and offering the reader the complete case histories of the 134 patients who were treated and whose outcome we had reported. We agreed that Dr Pauling would write about the nature of cancer and the effectiveness of megavitamin C therapy, discussions now included in the chapter "New Hope for Cancer Patients." He would also make the biostatistical analysis, while I was to prepare the clinical material, the case histories of my patients, and provide an analysis of the clinical data as a clinician. I insisted that Dr Pauling be named the first author of the book since the work originated because of his great interest in vitamin C and cancer, but he was determined that my name should appear first, presumably because I was the clinician of the team. I argued with him but he was adamant. I believe he did not want any one to think that he was taking credit for work done by someone else.

In spite of his immense prestige, Linus Pauling could not find a publisher who would publish our book. We should have anticipated this response because the Proceedings of the National Academy of Science,

Washington, had rejected our first paper. Eventually, I found a receptive publisher in Bob Hilderley who agreed to proceed, but by this time it was too late to have Dr Pauling participate in the final editing of the book, for he died soon after. After he died I assumed that I could still co-author this book with him, but certain complications made this impossible. Thus this book is mine alone in copyright, even though it is a collaborative work with Linus Pauling. I have included the material he wrote which was the final copy before going to press. I will indicate clearly the parts he contributed and the parts I have written. I invited Dr Zelek Herman, a colleague of Linus Pauling who had worked with him on the biostatistical analysis, to contribute an appendix explaining the methods Linus Pauling and he had worked on and how to apply this to evaluate cohorts of cancer patients.

Vitamins-as-Treatment Paradigm

When Professor Linus Pauling died 19 August 1994 at 93 years of age, he had become the most productive humanitarian scientist this world has ever seen. As a biochemist, peace activist, and orthomolecular scientist, his work was dedicated to discovering the molecular nature of man, ensuring the survival of our species, and preventing and treating disease – in sum, improving the quality of life. Perhaps only five scientists have made such an impact on our lives, an impact recognized in the two Nobel Prizes he received, for chemistry and for peace.

His research into the structure and interaction of molecules provided one cornerstone for modern chemistry and medicine. The development of modern complex molecules targeted for specific receptors would have been delayed even longer. He showed that genes were responsible for the structure of protein, following his classic work with the abnormal structure of the hemoglobin in sickle cell anemia. From this work he originated his concept of molecular medicine, which later became orthomolecular medicine and psychiatry, a field I had been exploring with my colleague Dr Humphry Osmond since the early 1950s while treating schizophrenia with megadoses of vitamin B-3 and vitamin C, a story told in my book *Vitamin B-3 & Schizophrenia: Discovery, Recovery, Controversy.*

During his prolonged campaign to ban atomic bomb testing, inspired by his understanding of the effects of radiation on our well being, Professor Pauling delivered over 500 lectures, an extraordinary effort that made him very unpopular with Western powers, including the United States and the Soviet Union, particularly Joseph Stalin, who denounced not only his peace activism but also his scientific discoveries. If not for his activism, Linus Pauling may have received a third Nobel Prize for being first to determine the double helix structure of DNA. The US State Department seized his passport once when he was planning to travel to England to attend an important international meeting in England where he would have gained the additional information he needed to deduce the correct chemical structure. Dr Crick, who shared the Nobel Prize for the discovery of the structure of the DNA molecule, stated that Linus Pauling had showed them how to solve the problem.

Dr Pauling's biochemical research and ethical beliefs converged in his work in orthomolecular medicine during the last 30 years of his life. Oddly, the entry of this double Nobel Prize winner into the field of medicine created a storm of opposition and criticism from the healing professions – physicians, psychiatrists, social workers, psychologists, nutritionists, and dietitians – as he argued that vitamins could be used therapeutically in optimum amounts or megadoses, not just in RDA doses, with no harm to one's health – in fact, with great beneficial effect on one's health. His books *Vitamin C and the Common Cold* and *How To Live Longer and Feel Better* were the flashpoints for one of the hottest controversies in medical history. Linus Pauling was not a trained medical doctor and his research was dismissed by the medical establishment as a result, odd since many of the world's most important medical discoveries have been made, not by medical doctors, but by inspired scientists like Louis Pasteur with his discovery that bacteria are involved in disease.

But even if he had been a medical doctor, Dr Pauling's work would have been opposed, as was our work with the treatment of schizophrenia, because he was thinking against the grain of established medical belief and practice. Dr Pauling had suddenly jumped from one paradigm of medical thought to another, from what I call the vitamin-as-prevention paradigm to the vitamin-as-treatment paradigm. Paradigm battles can be most ferocious. This is probably why it may take two generations, forty years, before a new idea is accepted into medicine.

The vitamin-as-prevention paradigm had been established by 1930 and has held sway into the 1990s, although the medical profession stoutly resisted it for many decades, refusing to believe that a disease could be produced by the absence of something. It was very useful in determining what vitamins were and the type of syndromes their absence generated. The *vitamin-as-prevention* paradigm includes this set of facts, more properly beliefs. (1) Vitamins are catalysts and therefore needed in minute quantities for the prevention of vitamin deficiency diseases such as beri beri (vitamin B-1), pellagra (vitamin B-3), and scurvy (vitamin C). Catalysts are not destroyed. They are simply re-used. (2) Therefore diseases not known as vitamin deficiency diseases should not be treated with vitamins. This follows the medical concept of one drug, one disease, or one vitamin, one deficiency disease. Using vitamins to treat non-deficiency diseases was considered unethical. Many physicians lost their license to practice because they violated this essential principle of this paradigm. In California, for example, it was considered malpractice to advise patients to take vitamin C if they had cancer. No one was allowed to tell their patients that the vitamin could be therapeutic. (3) Therefore doses above those recommended by food and drug administrations, the so-called RDA (Recommended Dietary Allowance) doses, are contra-indicated and even considered dangerous. Often where there is no toxicity it is invented – for example, the false belief that vitamin C will cause pernicious anemia because it destroys vitamin B-12 (it does not) or that vitamin C will cause kidney stones when it does not. This old paradigm became the bible for modern nutritionists and for the medical profession which had fled from any serious consideration of the importance of nutrition since about 1950, leaving the field to non-clinical dietitians and nutritionists, that is, to people who could not possibly use nutritional intervention as treatment and therefore could not see what nutrition or lack of nutrition could do. (4) A balanced diet will provide all the vitamins any one needs.

The roots of the vitamins-as-treatment paradigm can be traced to the 1940s when early pellagrologists discovered that chronic pellagrins required large doses of vitamin B-3 to remain free of pellagra. During the 1950s, Dr Humphry Osmond and I proved that large doses of vitamin B-3 were also effective in treating schizophrenia, a discovery first reported in the *Journal of Experimental Psychopathology* in 1957 and chronicled in my

Vitamin B-3 and Schizophrenia book published in 1998. While this research was largely ignored by the medical profession until the 1990s, our parallel discovery that niacin lowered serum cholesterol levels was the first major attack on the old paradigm to be accepted, but only after our findings were confirmed by W.B. Parsons and his colleagues at the Mayo Clinic. This finding is now recognized as the first introduction of the modern vitamin-as-treatment paradigm into accepted medical knowledge and practice. We used doses up to three grams daily, about 300 times the recommended daily requirement, to lower cholesterol levels. Hypercholesterolemia is not considered to be a vitamin deficiency disease.

The new paradigm, the *vitamins-as-treatment* paradigm, includes this set of facts. (1) Vitamins are needed not only for deficiency diseases but for other conditions as well, in optimum doses, not simply RDA doses, which may be small or large. There is no artificial restriction to only small doses. (2) Vitamins can be therapeutic for conditions not recognized as deficiencies – for example, niacin for decreasing cholesterol levels, where niacin is used in doses 300 times the RDA. (3) Vitamins, even in large doses, are safe, especially the water soluble ones. The toxicity of vitamins has been grossly exaggerated. (4) Very few people eat diets so well balanced they obtain adequate quantities of many of the vitamins, even when they are well. When they are under stress or ill, no diet is adequate without the supplementation of the important nutrients.

Paradigms in medicine and science are replaced by better ones as more information accrues. Additional facts can no longer be accounted for by the old paradigm and eventually directly contradict it. This topples the old paradigm. The battle may be long and ferocious, and even when it is generally replaced, there will remain a residue of fossilized scientists who will die swearing allegiance to it. Dr Pauling was a respected member of the old paradigm, but one day his faith in it was seriously challenged, and within a matter of days he had leapt from the old into the new, one of the first eminent scientists to make this quantum jump. Dr Pauling described how he became interested in megadose vitamin therapy many times. One afternoon he and Mrs Pauling were visiting a friend who had on her coffee table a copy of the book I had co-authored in 1966 with Dr Humphry Osmond, *How To Live With Schizophrenia*. The book had been given to her by the father of one of our patients who had recovered from her schizophrenia on a megavitamin regimen after five years of failure on standard treatment. Dr Pauling borrowed the book and spent that night reading it. He was not only surprised by the fact that we were using such high doses of vitamin B-3 and vitamin C with no harm to our patients, but also convinced by our reports on the efficacy of nutrient therapy, so much so that he postponed his retirement and began to champion the vitamin-as-treatment paradigm.

Dr Pauling's interest in vitamin therapy was a logical extension of his previous interest in molecular medicine, perhaps best stated in an address he gave to the California Institute of Technology, 16 May 1938, published later in *Science*, 1938. "Organic chemistry was developed into a great science during the nineteenth century," he stated, "and it seems probable that all or nearly all its fundamental principles have now been formulated. There is, however, a related field of knowledge of transcendent significance to mankind which has barely begun its development. This field deals with the correlation between chemical structure and physiological activity of those substances, manufactured in the body or ingested in foodstuffs, which are essential for orderly growth and the maintenance of life, as well as of the many substances which are useful in the treatment of disease." In 1968 Dr Pauling expanded this statement into the field of "orthomolecular" medicine, a term he coined to describe our work with vitamin B-3, vitamin C, and other nutrients in treating schizophrenics. In his report entitled "Orthomolecular Psychiatry" published in *Science*, Dr Pauling stated, "Orthomolecular therapy, consisting of the provision for the individual person of the optimum concentration of important normal constituents of the brain, may be the preferred treatment for many mentally ill patients." Elsewhere, he defined orthomolecular psychiatry as "the achievement and preservation of mental health by varying concentrations in the human body of substances that are normally present, such as vitamins. It is part of a broader subject, orthomolecular medicine, an important part because the functioning of the brain is probably more sensitively dependent on its molecular composition and structure than is the functioning of the organs."

Another colleague, Dr Bernard Rimland, author of *Infantile Autism*, further explains the meaning of orthomolecular and contrasts the practice of 'orthomolecular' medicine with 'toximolecular' medicine: "'Ortho' means straight or correct and 'molecular' refers to the chemistry of the body.

'Orthomolecular' thus means correcting the chemistry of the body. To contrast the philosophies of establishment medicine and orthomolecular medicine, I have coined the word 'toximolecular' to refer to the common practice of trying to treat disease (or at least the symptoms of disease) through the use of toxic chemicals. It doesn't make much sense to me; it is dangerous, expensive, and not very effective. But it is profitable. Most vitamins are quite safe, in contrast to the drugs in widespread use which can be and all too often are lethal in large amounts. Traditional medicine consists largely of giving lethal drugs in sub-lethal amounts, it seems to me. Orthomolecular psychiatry is not only much safer, it is much more sensible. Its emphasis on the use of substances normally present in the human really makes sense."

The practice of orthomolecular medicine thus recognizes that most acute and chronic diseases are due to a metabolic fault which is correctable in most patients by good nutrition, including the use of large doses of vitamins and mineral supplements. In sharp contrast, drugs are synthetics which are not naturally present in the body and for which the body does not have ready made mechanisms for their destruction and elimination. They are called xenobiotics – that is, foreign molecules. And unlike conventional medicine, orthomolecular medicine recognizes the principle of individuality in recommending the optimum diet of nutrients for each of us. No two patients are the same; no two treatments are the same. Orthomolecular medicine requires the application of both these principles, individuality and the use of optimum doses (large doses if needed) of vitamins, minerals, amino and essential fatty acids.

Dr Pauling became very supportive of the work being done by our colleagues, and within a few years we agreed that we were in fact practicing orthomolecular psychiatry and that we should officially adopt this term as representative of what we were doing. In 1973 Dr Pauling co-edited with David Hawkins a book called *Orthomolecular Psychiatry* which was instigated by The Committee on Therapy of the American Schizophrenia Association, which I chaired at the time. By now Dr Pauling was fully identified with the new paradigm and with orthomolecular psychiatry and medicine. In 1971 he established the Linus Pauling Institute of Science and Medicine to study orthomolecular medicine, especially the relation of vitamin B-3 and vitamin C to schizophrenia. Dr Pauling's efforts delighted those of us who were practicing megavitamin therapy with these two and with other vitamins, but excited a tremendous amount of hostility and criticism from the psychiatric profession. The American Psychiatric Association tried to suppress the publication of any information about the value of high dose vitamins in the treatment of schizophrenia. They eventually called Dr Osmond and me before their committee on ethics in 1971 because a California psychiatrist had complained about my paper describing the patient who recovered and whose father had indirectly introduced Dr Pauling to our concepts. Had the APA had their way, Dr Pauling might not have seen our work and his interest might have been mislaid or delayed.

During this time, Dr Pauling met Dr Irwin Stone, who had argued in a number of articles that megadoses of vitamin C were effective for treating the common cold and for improving health in general. Dr Stone had been taking ascorbic acid himself, 3 grams daily, and in response to a comment Dr Pauling made in a public lecture expressing his desire to live for another 25 years so he could witness and participate in more scientific discoveries, Dr Stone assured him he could achieve his wish by taking megadoses of ascorbic acid. (Incidentally, Dr Pauling did live another 30 years after beginning to take vitamin C, and Dr Stone invented the term "megadose" as applied to vitamins, not I, as some believe.) Dr Stone's book *The Healing Factor: Vitamin C against Disease* and Dr Pauling's *Vitamin C and the Common Cold* first made the vitamins-as-treatment paradigm public in the early 1970s.

In an address in 1991 to the "Second World Congress on Vitamin C and the Immune System," Dr Pauling told this story about his meeting with Dr Stone, his subsequent 'conversion' to the vitamin-as-treatment paradigm, and the resulting controversy as he championed this attitude against such cancer establishment doctors as Victor Herbert and others who tried to discredit his research. "When Irvine Stone wrote to me in 1965, after having heard me give a talk in which I said that I would like to live 25 years longer in order to enjoy reading about the new discoveries about the nature of the world that no doubt would be made by scientists during these 25 years, and said if I were to take 3 grams a day of vitamin C, I would perhaps not only live the 25 years but even 50 years, that was when I increased my uptake of ascorbate fifty-fold to 3,000 milligrams a day, then later to a hundred-fold, 6,000 milligrams, then to two-hundred-fold, then to three-hundred-fold

– and I'm still not sure what the optimum intake is. There is a practical reason why I stopped at three-hundred-fold, at 18,000 milligrams. Well, I think that's pretty important. I read a statement by physicians that they should tell their patients not to worry about being constipated. I think they should worry about being constipated: it's so harmful to carry waste toxic materials around for an unnecessarily long period of time. So, it was Irwin Stone that got me interested in vitamin C and, of course, it was that scoundrel Victor Herbert who was responsible for my having begun writing books about vitamins.

"So the other day I received a book published by the National Academy of Sciences on control of diseases. It mentions practically nothing about vitamins and their usefulness but does have something about common colds, a statement that 16 control trials have been turned out, every one of which showed that vitamin C has no value in preventing or controlling the common cold. I'm sure they're the 16 control trials that I discuss in my books, where I give the amount of decrease in illness. Every one of these trials shows that vitamin C has value, not that it doesn't have value. That's perhaps a minor misrepresentation. A couple of years ago, I got two or three letters from people who sent me clippings from a magazine discrediting my work. One of them said he had stopped taking his vitamin C because of the statement in this magazine, featuring a quotation from a noted professor of medicine at Yale University Medical School advising that you shouldn't take as much as even one gram of vitamin C per day because it will damage the liver. So I wrote to this professor and said that I read the literature on vitamin C to the extent that I can – there are a couple of thousand new papers published every year about vitamin C. 'Would you please send me the references to the work done on the damage done to the liver,' I asked. Well, he was a gentleman, which you'd expect at Yale Medical School, though often when I write letters like that I don't get an answer. He wrote back saying, 'Oh, that was just a mistake.' That was the end of that. So far as I know he didn't write to the magazine and say that was a mistake, but he did say it to me. And there are lots of mistakes of this sort about vitamins that perhaps sometimes intentionally misrepresent the facts. For some perhaps there is an economic or financial reason. There is so much opposition in the medical establishment against improving your health by taking vitamins."

A few years after publishing *Vitamin C and the Common Cold*, Dr Pauling became interested in anti-cancer potential of vitamin C. In an address to the newly-opened Ben May Institute, he suggested that vitamin C might be useful in the treatment of cancer. But Dr Victor Herbert, one of his most severe critics, was extremely critical of this statement, which challenged Dr Pauling to examine the literature and thereby to meet Dr Ewan Cameron who was using vitamin C in treating his terminal cancer patients. In 1979 Dr Cameron and Linus Pauling published their book *Cancer and Vitamin C*, which was revised in 1993 and augmented with a report on my work with cancer patients using megavitamin therapy. This book is primarily an account of the results of clinical studies conducted by Dr Cameron in Scotland at the Vales of Leven hospital where megadoses of vitamin C were given to patients suffering from a variety of cancers. As of 10 August 1976 all of the 1,000 control patients, those who did not receive vitamin C therapy, were dead, while 18 of the 100 treated with vitamin C were still alive. The mean time of survival for the treated group was 4.2 times as great as it was for the control group. They lived more than 300 days longer. As Dr John Hoffer concluded in a review of this study, "the favorable effect of vitamin C in the Vale of Leven cancer patients, while not excellent, was far from negligible. Indeed it was comparable to the effect reported for IL-2 in later NCI-funded Phase II trials that attracted wide interest in the scientific medical community. Most important from the biologic perspective were the cases in which vitamin C induced catastrophic tumor hemorrhage and necrosis. Although IL-2 occasionally produces rapid remissions, it has never had an effect as dramatic as this." However, the Cameron-Pauling studies were perceived by the 'cancer establishment' as an attack on the common cancer treatment paradigm and therefore were totally unacceptable.

Cancer and Vitamin C was highly controversial among the profession, where this report was denounced in two articles from the Mayo Clinic published in the *New England Journal of Medicine*, but also inspirational for me because by chance I had already seen what a combination of vitamin B-3 and vitamin C had done to a few patients with terminal cancer. And so began my clinical study of this form of orthomolecular therapy, the source of the information presented in this book.

Dr Linus Pauling was a great teacher, a brilliant investigator, a sensitive and honest colleague, and a great humanitarian. The foundation he laid for orthomolecular medicine will never be forgotten, and the work he started has gained a momentum so great that it can no longer be hindered or stopped. A scientist will be judged not only by the validity of his work and by the opinion of his peers but also by the quality of his enemies and critics. Professor Linus Pauling had innumerable friends and supporters among my colleagues and among the lay public, but his critics were few, though highly influential. As listed in the news reports following his death, they included Joseph McCarthy, Senator from Wisconsin, Chairman of the Senate Permanent Committee on Investigations, who labeled him a communist which prompted The State Department to revoke his passport in 1952; Joseph Stalin, who considered him hostile to Marxist views and condemned his theory of resonance of molecules as pseudo- scientific; Dr Arthur Robinson, a former colleague and supporter, who accused him of suppressing his research because it did not agree with Dr Pauling's view on ascorbic acid and cancer and who accused him of hurting his wife who had cancer by giving her vitamin C; Dr Victor Herbert, who maintained that Dr Pauling was psychotic about vitamin C, calling him "delusional" on a CBC-TV program, where he contended that Dr Pauling would shorten his life by taking vitamin C, adding that had Dr Pauling not taken any vitamin C he would live to age 105.

A few months before his death, I participated in a conference in San Francisco on "Therapeutic Potential of Biological Antioxidants," sponsored by the Linus Pauling Institute of Science and Medicine. Dr Pauling had been asked that he record a statement to this meeting in the event that he died before it was held. He refused to do so, believing firmly he would be able to deliver it himself. As I listened to the various speakers, from about 20 universities around the world, I suddenly realized that a meeting on this subject with these participants could not have been held if Dr Pauling had retired at age 65 when he first contemplated doing so and had not become the champion of orthomolecular medicine. Tribute was paid to Dr Pauling by scientists from around the world, from France, from Croatia, from South America, as well as from the United States and Canada.

Complementary Therapy

Despite the fears of some critics, this book is not an attack on the medical profession and the use of the standard methods for treating cancer, which include surgery, radiation, and chemotherapy. Rather, we have attempted to redress the imbalance that exists today between these xenobiotic or drug treatments and nutritional or orthomolecular therapy. This therapy is not an 'alternative' in the sense that it insists standard methods must not be used. The therapy recommended is 'complementary' in the sense that the best of both xenobiotic and nutritional or orthomolecular medicine should be used, individualized for each patient by the doctors advising and treating the patients.

We need to redress the imbalance. No reasonable person can argue that the cancer situation today is very good. Surely after the expenditure of billions of dollars on one approach which has been rarely successful when used alone, it is imperative that other approaches be examined. It is necessary to let the public know that complementary treatment is available and to alert the press that they should pay as much attention to the newer developments in this field as they do to the standard approaches. It is an attempt to bring nutrition back into medicine, restoring the role it played for hundreds of years.

– Abram Hoffer

1 NEW HOPE FOR CANCER PATIENTS

There is now much reason for people with cancer to hope that they can overcome the disease and live good lives extending to the normal life span. Even patients who are judged by their physicians to have reached the "terminal" or "untreatable" stage of their disease (untreatable by conventional methods) no longer need to be despondent; instead, they should recognize that changes in their lifestyles, especially in their nutrition, can be decisive in checking and even reversing the progress of their malignancies. This is the message of this book.

We have reached this opinion through the consideration of clinical studies and of progress in the scientific study of cancer and of nutrition, especially of vitamins, during the past quarter century. Although the evidence for this opinion has not yet been accepted by the medical establishment, a good number of physicians in the United States, Canada, Scotland, the Netherlands, Germany, Switzerland, and other countries are making use of the regimen that we describe in this book, as a adjunct to appropriate conventional treatment (if any is known).

Beginning about 50 years ago, shortly after vitamin supplements became available, physicians began publishing their observations that patients with cancer seemed to benefit from the daily intake of large amounts, usually 1,000 to 2,000 milligrams, of vitamin C, often together with large amounts of vitamin A. These early reports were summarized by Irwin Stone in his book *The Healing Factor: Vitamin C against Disease.* Little attention was paid to these reports, however, until Dr Ewan Cameron during the 1970s began giving patients with advanced ("untreatable") cancer in Vale of Leven Hospital, Lochlomondside, Scotland, a course of 10,000 milligrams per day of sodium ascorbate by intravenous infusion for two weeks in addition to 10,000 milligrams per day taken by mouth and continued indefinitely. He found that this regimen improved the quality of life and greatly extended the survival times of the patients. His efforts since then to have vitamin C used by the established medical community as an adjunct to appropriate conventional therapy have, nevertheless, met with only limited response until now.

The Nature of Cancer

Since the development of molecular biology, beginning about 50 years ago, the understanding of the nature and causes of cancer has been increasing rapidly. The nature of every cell in the body of a human being is primarily determined by the genetic material – DNA (deoxyribonucleic acid), mostly in the chromosomes) – that the person has inherited from his or her parents. Over the many millions of years of evolution the genetic material has changed, but for each surviving species it has such a composition as to keep the individuals of the species alive and in sufficiently good health to permit them to become adults and to produce offspring, who constitute the next generation, which is necessary if the species is not to die out. For homo sapiens this process has continued for 200,000 years, leading to modern humans, who reach puberty in their middle teens. Technically, about 15 years is required to produce the next generation. We can accordingly understand why good health generally continues until about age 20. This age was, in fact, the probable life expectancy for stone-age man, and even later, through the classical period and the middle ages.

The evolutionary process ignored the health of human beings after the necessary period of procreation. We can accordingly understand why after age 30 the chance of dying doubles with every increase of 8 years in chronological age, being 64 times as great at age 78 as at age 30.

One aspect of aging is that the thousands of biochemical reactions, such as those involved in burning glucose and other fuels to provide heat and energy, do not proceed as fast in old people as in younger ones. Part of the process of aging consists of a decrease in the amounts of enzymes produced in the cell, which are themselves becoming aged. Most of the biochemical reactions make use of enzymes, with vitamins and the essential metals as coenzymes, in speeding up the biochemical reactions, and the reactions can be made to go faster by providing more of these important nutrients. This argument provides a strong basis for increasing the intake of the nutrients with increase in age. It is now generally accepted that a cancer results from a change in the genetic material in a cell, which then grows out of control. The change may be any one of several kinds. The most common one is the replacement of one base pair (one nucleotide in each of the two DNA strands in the double helix) by another. Such a change (a mutation) may cause the cell to divide steadily to produce a cluster of similar cells, a swelling, that is called a tumor. If the tumor does infiltrate (invade) the neighboring tissues and does not metastasize to other parts of the body, it is called a benign tumor, usually offering little danger, but if it has the powers of infiltration and metastasis, it is called a malignant tumor, a cancer.

During the 1970s it was discovered that there are certain genes (DNA sequences) normally present in the human genome (total DNA of one human) that undergo mutations which change the normal cell into a malignant cell. These genes are called oncogenes, from the Greek word *oncos*, meaning a mass or tumor. Accordingly, an oncologist is a physician who specializes in cancer.

The mutation leading to malignancy may be caused by high-energy radiation, by long exposure to increased heat (as in the lips of pipe smokers), by repeated mechanical effects (the lips of trumpet players), by entry of a virus into a cell, or by exposure to chemicals. Hundreds of chemicals are known to be carcinogenic.

But why do cancers develop in some people but not in others?

Dr Rene Dobos, the microbiologist at the Rockefeller Institute for Medical Research who discovered the first antibiotics to be used in the control of disease (gramicidine and tyrocidin), said that viruses and bacteria do not cause an infectious disease, but that the disease is caused by the person who contracts it. He was impressed by the fact that during an epidemic of viral or bacterial disease some people become sick and die, whereas others remain well. He knew, of course, that the virus or bacterium is involved in the disease. He was, however, emphasizing the fact that for some exposed people the natural protective mechanisms of the human body function so well as to prevent the disease from developing and for others these mechanisms function less well – and the people become sick and may die.

Dr Cameron, now Medical Director of the Linus Pauling Institute of Science and Medicine, has pointed out that when surgical removal of a malignant tumor is carried out, millions of malignant cells are released into the blood stream. Some of these migrant cells may settle down in some parts of the body to cause new malignant tumors of the same kind as the primary tumor; they are called metastatic tumors or metastases. For some patients, though, no metastases develop. It is reasonable to conclude that the natural protective mechanisms are more effective for the patients who do not develop metastases than for the others. It is indeed known that the immune mechanism of the human body can identify malignant cells and can then destroy them, and it is known that patients whose immune mechanisms are working well have a smaller chance of developing metastases than patients with deficient immune systems.

These and other similar facts support the conclusion that the risk of contracting cancer and dying of the disease is determined to some extent by the nature and condition of the body of the person, which are themselves determined by many factors. A very important one is the person's genotype, inherited directly from the parents and indirectly from the earlier ancestors. For example, the male descendants of Queen Victoria who carried the gene for hemophilia (the failure of blood to clot) tended to have this disease. In some families there is a genetic factor tending to the development of certain kinds of cancer and in others there are factors making the immune system strong or weak.

Why do some patients die and others survive? Several possible reasons have already been mentioned. The difference between the two kinds of patients may be the result of their different heredities, about which little can now be done. Patients with a well-functioning immune system have a better prognosis than those with a weak immune system, and there are known treatments with substances that stimulate the immune system (immunostimulants), some of which are used to some extent, but not widely, in conventional cancer therapy, and others that are used in unconventional cancer therapy. Nutrients, including vitamins, are important in bolstering the immune system.

Other factors affecting the risk of developing cancer and of dying from the disease are environmental. For example, children who were exposed to x-rays before they were born, when x-ray photographs were made of the pelvic regions of their mothers, tend to develop cancer. Skin cancers tend to form when the skin has too much exposure to sunlight. The radioactive fission products and Carbon 14 from the testing of nuclear weapons and from nuclear power plant disasters such as Three Mile Island and Chernobyl are causing many people all over the world to develop cancer and also causing many infants to be born with gross physical and mental defects who otherwise would have been normal. High-energy radiation causes the formation of free radicals, which are believed to be responsible for its harmful effects, and, indeed, partially responsible for the changes in the human body called aging. Free radicals are molecules from which an electron has been knocked out or to which an extra electron has been added, making it especially active in attacking the genetic material (DNA) and other molecules in the body and in this way causing cancer and doing other damage.

But man-made high-energy radiation is not the only producer of free radicals. Every person is continually being exposed to natural high-energy radiation, consisting of cosmic rays, radiation from outer space that reaches the surface of the earth, and natural radioactivity, especially a radioactive form of potassium that is present everywhere, radium in rocks, and the radioactive gas radon that is present in the air, in larger amounts in high-radium regions.

The human body attempts to protect itself against free radicals. For example, every cell in the body contains a large number of molecules or a special protein called superoxide dismutase. This protein is an enzyme, a molecule that has the property of speeding up certain biochemical reactions, in this case the destruction of a particular free radical called the superoxide radical. The destruction of free radicals also requires certain substances called antioxidants. It was shown recently in 1989 by B. Frei and associates that the most important antioxidant is vitamin C, followed by vitamin E. We may conclude accordingly that some added protection against cancer and some slowing down of the aging process can be achieved by increasing the intake of these vitamins.

Many substances (often called chemicals) are known to cause cancer. Some of these substances occur in nature. For example, Aspergillus fungus growing on moldy grains and peanut meal produces toxic compounds of carbon, oxygen, and hydrogen, called aflatoxins, that are very carcinogenic, causing cancer of the liver in human beings. Care must be taken to keep aflatoxins out of peanut butter. Also, nitrates and nitrites, sometimes present naturally in foods or used in their preparation, as in the curing of bacon, cause cancer of the esophagus. During recent years it has been shown that an increased intake of vitamin C tends to prevent these carcinogenic effects of toxic substances.

In addition to the natural carcinogenic agents, there are also present in the environment others that are produced by man. Thousands of toxic chemicals are now being made, some of them in amounts of hundreds of tons per year. Among them are the insecticides and other pesticides that are used in agriculture. The toxic substances in cigarette smoke cause about one quarter of the deaths by cancer in the United States. The carcinogenicity of substances can be determined by study of animals and of humans with unusually large exposures to the substances. Governments of many countries try to prevent the manufacture and use of those found to be carcinogenic. This effort has been only partially successful. One of the functions of vitamin C in the human body is in helping to destroy toxic substances, converting them into innocuous substances that are then eliminated in the urine. This fact provides additional evidence to support the message of this book.

Not every person who is exposed to a carcinogenic agent develops cancer, and not every person who develops cancer dies of this disease. In the United States, about 800,000 people per year are newly diagnosed as having developed cancer (not including the common form of skin cancer, basal cell carcinoma, usually caused by excessive exposure to the sun, which is easy to cure and rarely leads to death). Only about 450,000 of these people die of cancer, however, so that nearly one half of these cancer patients survive, and may be said to have been cured by their treatment or to have experienced a spontaneous recovery. This fact – that many cancer patients survive – can give everyone cause for hope. This knowledge of the antioxidant and antitoxic properties of vitamin C is supported by the clinical observations reported in this book, based on the treatment of 134 patients with advanced cancer and with psychiatric problems (mainly severe depression and anxiety) who were registered with Dr Abram Hoffer by referral from a primary physician during a dozen years ending 15 April 1989 (the close of the study), and on a series of follow-up studies conducted by Dr Hoffer from 1989-1996. These patients were treated for their psychiatric problems in the same way as other psychiatric patients without cancer. This treatment, used by Dr Hoffer for about 40 years, involved the daily intake of mega amounts of vitamin C, vitamin B-3, vitamin E, and several other nutrients. After some time, Dr Hoffer noticed that the cancer patients following his regimen, and in some cases also receiving some conventional treatment, seemed clearly to be living longer than expected.

Most of the evidence discussed in this book relates to the effectiveness of megavitamins in the treatment of patients with advanced cancer. Our conclusion is that about 50 percent of these patients with advanced cancer can be "cured" (survival for over five years). We surmise that if the megavitamin regimen were to be started at the time of first diagnosis of cancer, as an adjunct to appropriate conventional therapy, the cancer death rate could be reduced to 25 percent of its present value, and moreover, if, in the course of time, a reasonable megavitamin regimen were to be followed regularly by every person, as a way of improving the health and decreasing the incidence of cancer and other diseases, the cancer death rate would fall to one eighth of its present value.

With the usual classification of diseases, cancer is the next to leading cause of death in the United States after diseases of the heart, accounting for 19 percent of all deaths in 1990, a total 440,000 lives. If the cancer death rate fell to one eighth of this total, 385,000 lives would be saved.

Nutritional or Orthomolecular Medicine

Nutrients are the constituents of foods that provide nourishment to a human being or other animal. During the 19th century, it was found that the major nutrients are the fats, the carbohydrates, the proteins, and water. It was then discovered that there are other nutrients, present in rather small amounts in food, that are required for good health and for life. It had, in fact, been known since antiquity that common salt, sodium chloride, is needed, and also it was learned in the 17th century that bones contain phosphorus as well as calcium, so that compounds of these elements are needed for the development of bones. In 1881 the Swiss biochemist Lunin found that mice died when they were fed a mixture of purified fat, carbohydrate, protein, and minerals, but survived if a little milk was added to the diet. Many such studies during the next 50 years led to the identification of the vitamins, essential fats, and other important nutrients that are present in foods in small amounts and that contribute to good health, some of them being required for life.

Fats, Carbohydrates, and Proteins

The fats are colorless and odorless greasy substances that are the chief constituents of the fatty tissues of animals and are also found in plants. Lard, the nearly pure fat from pigs, is white, but tallow, from cows, is pale yellow because of impurities. The Roman author Pliny the Elder wrote in about 50 A.D. that the Germans were making a soap solution by boiling fat with the ashes of plants (potash). In 1779 the Swedish chemist K.W. Scheele discovered that this soap solution contains not only soap, the potassium salt of a fatty acid, but also an oily, sweet-tasting, water-soluble liquid that we now call glycerine or glycerol. The French chemist Michel Chevreul then showed in 1820 that the fats consist of molecules of glycerol, each combined with three residues of fatty acid, which may differ from one another in the length of the chains of carbon atoms and the number of double bonds. A fat containing fatty acids with no double bonds is said to be saturated, with a few double bonds unsaturated, and with many double bonds polyunsaturated. The saturated fats are solid at room temperature; the unsaturated and polyunsaturated fat (oils) are liquid.

The constituent of blood reported by a laboratory as "triglyceride" is fat. Fat is an important constituent of a good diet in several ways. It provides the fat-soluble vitamins, the essential fatty acids, and other fat-soluble nutrients such as coenzyme Q and lecithin. It is also an important source of bodily energy.

The carbohydrates are compounds of carbon, hydrogen, and oxygen in the same ratio as in water, H_2O. The important simple carbohydrates are glucose and fructose, both $C_6H_{12}O_6$, and sucrose, $C_{12}H_{22}O_{11}$. Sucrose, ordinary sugar, is the condensation product of glucose and fructose which are bonded together with elimination of one water molecule. These simple sugars are found especially in fruits and honey. Starch, the most important carbohydrate in foods, consists of very large molecules that are composed of glucose residues. When starch is digested, it adds water to form glucose, which enters the blood stream, later to be oxidized to water and carbon dioxide in the muscle cells and other cells to provide energy for muscular work and for fueling other biochemical reactions that require energy.

At the present time, about 20 percent of our food energy in the typical North American and European diet is provided by starch, about 6 percent by glucose and fructose from fruits and honey, and about 20 percent from sucrose, most of which is pure sucrose added to foods and drinks from the sugar bowl or in the process of preparation. A high intake of sucrose is associated with high incidence of cardiovascular disease.

The proteins constitute a group consisting of billions of similar substances present in living organisms. The molecules are very large; for example, the molecule of human hemoglobin, the red protein in the red cells in the blood, consists of about 10,000 atoms. Each human being may have as many as 50,000 different kinds of protein in the body. Animals of different species, with rare exceptions, make different kinds of protein. It was discovered about 150 years ago that when a protein is boiled in an acidic or basic solution, it is broken down into substances with smaller molecules, and it is now known that proteins are composed of about 20 different groups called amino acid residues, which are linked together into chains (polypeptide chains). A protein molecule may consist of a single chain, say of 150 residues, as in myoglobin (the oxygen carrying protein in human muscle), or of several chains, 4 in human hemoglobin.

Many protein molecules also have other atoms or groups of atoms attached to the polypeptide chains. In both myoglobin and hemoglobin, there is such a group (one per chain), a group that contains an iron atom that has the function of hooking on to an oxygen molecule in the lungs and then later releasing it. In this way hemoglobin carries oxygen from the lungs to the tissue, where it diffuses through the walls of the blood capillaries and is picked up by the myoglobin and transported to the muscle cells.

Proteins are present in both plant and animal foods. Digestion of proteins splits them into the amino acids, which go through the walls of the intestines, enter the blood stream, and are taken to the cells throughout the body. There they are combined in many new ways, characteristic of the individual human being, as determined by his inherited DNA templates.

Protein molecules are continually being broken down in the body, and are converted to water, carbon dioxide, and urea. A supply of new protein is constantly needed. These molecules are synthesized in the cells from the amino acids that have been derived from the digestion of the proteins in the ingested food. Careful studies have shown that the amount of ordinary food protein required each day for this replenishment is a little less than half a gram per kilogram body weight for an adult (more is needed for an infant or growing child or teenager). This comes to 35 grams (1.25 ounces) per day for a 70 kilogram (154 pound) adult. The present American diet provides about twice this amount. Protein starvation is rare in the United States but common in some underdeveloped countries.

Water is an essential nutrient. A high intake leads to good health and helps in preventing kidney disease and gout and perhaps arthritis.

It was discovered around 1840 that energy cannot be created or destroyed – the law of conservation of energy. Later it was found that matter can be converted into energy and energy into matter, the amounts being related by the Einstein equation $E = mc^2$, in which E is the amount of energy, m is the mass and c^2 is the square of the velocity of light. This interconversion of matter and energy is important in radioactivity and in the reactions that keep the sun hot, but not in the functioning of living organisms. The energy that keeps a person warm and permits him or her to do work is provided by the oxidation of foods, mainly the fats, carbohydrates, and proteins, in the cells of the body.

Fats provide about 900 kcal per 100 grams, carbohydrates about 410 kcal per 100 grams, and proteins about 430 kcal per 100 grams. The kilocalorie (kcal) is the amount of energy required to raise the temperature of l kilogram (2.2 pounds) of water by 1°Celsius (1.8°F). A person of ordinary size doing a moderate amount of physical work might require about 2400 kcal per day, which could be provided by a daily diet containing about 110 grams (4 ounces) of fat, 300 grams (11 ounces) of carbohydrate, and 60 grams (2 ounces) of protein. Intake of much larger amounts of food than needed leads to obesity, especially in persons with an inherited tendency to store fat in the adipose tissues.

The energy distribution among fats, carbohydrates, and proteins in the average American diet is given in Table 1, with the dietary goals of the nation, established in "Dietary Goals for the United States" by the Senate Select Committee on Nutrition and Human Needs, 1976.

Vitamins and Minerals

A vitamin is defined as an organic compound (a compound containing carbon atoms) found in human food of plant and animal origin and essential to human health and life. Vitamins may be obtained from foods or from nutritional supplements (vitamin tablets). A deficiency in the intake of a vitamin leads to disease and, if continued, may result in death.

The common vitamin-deficiency diseases are scurvy (deficiency in vitamin C, ascorbic acid or ascorbate), beri beri (deficiency in thiamine, vitamin B-1), night-blindness and other problems (deficiency in vitamin A),

TABLE 1

Energy Distribution of Average USA Diet vs USA Dietary Goals

	Diet	Goal		
Fat	42%	30%	40%	(1000 kcal/day)
Protein	12%	12%	10%	(250 kcal/day)
Carbohydrate	46%	58%	50%	(1250kcal/day)
Starch	20%	38%	38%	
Natural Sugars	6%	10%	10%	
Sucrose	20%	10%	10%	
Total	100%	200%	100%	(2500kcal/day)

rickets (deficiency in vitamin D), pellagra (deficiency in vitamin B-3, niacin or niacinamide), and pernicious anemia (deficiency in vitamin B-12, cyanocobalamin). Some of these diseases, especially scurvy and beri beri, caused a tremendous amount of suffering before the vitamins were discovered.

During the last 50 years a great deal of effort has been made to determine the daily intakes of vitamins and minerals needed to prevent, in most people in ordinary health, the overt occurrence of the corresponding deficiency diseases. These efforts have been successful. The daily amounts needed are called the RDAs (recommended dietary allowances). Table 2 suggests values for American people from the 1989 report of the Food and Nutrition Board of the National Academy of Sciences.

Although the RDAs can be accepted as the daily amounts that for most people prevent the development of obvious deficiency diseases, they are not the "optimum dietary allowances" that lead to the best of health and make the maximum contribution to the prevention and treatment of disease in general, including cancer and cardiovascular diseases.

The word megavitamin comes from the Greek word megas, meaning large or great. Scientists use the prefix mega to mean one million; thus a one-megaton nuclear warhead has explosive power equal to that of a million tons of TNT or dynamite. A megavitamin, however, is defined in terms of the dosage in which the vitamin is to be taken; a megavitamin intake is much larger than the RDA, not a million times, but usually in the range 25 to 1,000 times as great.

I first became aware of the megavitamins in April 1966 when I received a letter from a biochemist, Irwin Stone, who had heard me give a talk in New York in which I mentioned having been suffering from a cold and also said that I hope to live 25 years longer in order to have the pleasure of

TABLE 2

Recommended Dietary Allowances for a Few Vitamins in mg.

	B-1	B-2	B-3	B-6	C	E
Males	1.5	1.7	19	2.0	60	10
Females	1.1	1.3	15	1.6	60	8

learning about all the new discoveries that scientists would be continuing to make. He wrote that if I were to take 3,000 milligrams of vitamin C each day, I would not suffer severely from colds and that I might well live 50 years longer, not just 25. He sent me copies of his published papers, in which he gave several reasons for believing that the optimum daily intake of vitamin C is not 50 milligrams per day (the RDA) but far greater.

Vitamin C differs from all the other vitamins in that only a few species of animals require it as a vitamin. Human beings, cows, horses, mice, rats, guinea pigs, and all other mammals (also fish and reptiles) all require vitamin A, vitamin B-1, and vitamin C. These species have lost the ability to make these vitamins themselves, even though their ancestors likely could by eating plants, which manufacture all of these substances, and hence derive from their food enough vitamins to satisfy their needs to the extent sufficient to keep them alive long enough to have progeny, without the need for them to use energy and material to make additional amounts of these substances. Only a few species of animals have lost this ability.

Because of this loss, these animals must get vitamin C as ascorbate or ascorbic acid in their food or as a nutritional supplement. The guinea pig is such an animal. Accordingly, the companies that make food for the guinea pig add vitamin C to it, as well as the other vitamins, whereas they add only the other vitamins, not vitamin C, to the foods for cats, dogs, hamsters, and other animals, all of which are able to make their own vitamin C. An exception is the monkey which cannot synthesize vitamin C, and accordingly a good amount is added to monkey chow, in order to keep the laboratory monkeys in good health. In fact, all of the primates, including the anthropoid apes and human beings, have lost the ability to synthesize this vitamin. This loss presumably occurred in the common ancestor of the primates, about 40 million years ago.

Because of the importance of keeping laboratory monkeys in good health, careful studies have been made of the health of monkeys in relation to their daily intake of vitamin C. As a result of these studies, the chow for monkeys provides a far larger amount of this vitamin than the RDA for humans, roughly 50 times as much. This fact suggests that the optimum daily intake for humans might well be a megavitamin amount of this vitamin, perhaps 2,500 milligrams instead of the RDA of 60 milligrams.

As was emphasized by Irwin Stone in his scientific articles and his 1972 book *The Healing Factor: Vitamin C against Disease*, these facts and others strongly indicate that the optimum daily intake of vitamin C is a megavitamin amount, between 2,500 and 20,000 milligrams, and even more for people suffering from a disease. Irwin Stone emphasized in 1965 that almost every human being is suffering from this one important genetic vitamin deficiency disease, which he called hypoascorbemia (too small an amount of vitamin C in the blood). There is also evidence for the value of megavitamin amounts of other vitamins. It may well be that nearly every human being is suffering from several other diseases, the result of not ingesting regularly the optimum amounts of several other vitamins. Care must be taken, however, not to overdo the fat-soluble vitamins, A, D, and K. There is, however, no significant toxicity of megadoses (such as 800 IU) of vitamin E. Care must also be taken with the minerals; usually the optimum intake for them is close to the RDA.

About the same time that Irwin Stone wrote to me in 1965, I happened to read several papers and a book by Abram Hoffer and his associate Humphry Osmond about their observations that vitamin B-3 and vitamin C have value in the treatment of schizophrenic patients. I had been carrying on research on the molecular basis of mental disease since 1963, and I knew that several vitamins and many other substances are normally present in the brain and seem to be required for its proper functioning, and also that other substances can damage the brain and can cause mental illness. What astonished me was that Hoffer and Osmond were giving patients daily doses of vitamin B-3 and vitamin C hundreds or even thousands of times as much as their RDAs, without producing signs of toxicity. This extraordinary low toxicity clearly differentiates these vitamins from drugs, which are dangerously toxic and even lethal when taken in doses a few times large than those prescribed for the treatment of disease. I recognized also that many substances that are normally present in the human body and that are not vitamins also have low toxicity. These facts suggested to me that these substances should have a name, and I decided to call them "orthomolecular" substances. The prefix ortho is from the Greek work *orthos*, meaning right or correct. Vitamins are in this class of substances.

Orthomolecular medicine is the prevention or treatment of disease by regulating the concentrations in the human body of orthomolecular substances. My first use of the word was in my presidential address to the

Society on Vital Substances and the Diseases of Civilization on 18 September 1967 entitled "Orthomolecular Somatic and Psychiatric Medicine," followed in 1968 by a paper on "Orthomolecular Psychiatry" in the journal *Science.*

An example of orthomolecular medicine is the control of the genetic disease phenylketonuria, characterized by the presence of too high a concentration of the amino acid phenylalanine in the blood, by the provision from an early age (two months) of a special diet low in phenylalanine. Another example is the control of diabetes by the injection of insulin. Hundreds of diseases are now known to be controllable by orthomolecular methods, often by the provision of mega amounts of a vitamin.

The biochemist and nutritionist Roger J. Williams, who discovered the vitamin pantothenic acid and was one of the founders of the modern science of nutrition, emphasized in his teaching that human beings differ from one another in their biochemistry and in their nutritional needs. Some people have a genetic abnormality such that their need for a particular vitamin or other nutrient is especially great. For example, some people develop the carpal tunnel syndrome, in which the nerves in the wrists are compressed, crippling the hands. The regular intake of megadoses (100 times the RDA, or even more) of vitamin B-6 (pyridoxine) controls this disease in many patients.

It is now clear that there are two important daily intakes for each vitamin. One is the RDA, the intake recommended by the Food and Nutrition Board of the U.S. National Academy of Sciences, the amount considered to be enough to prevent obvious signs of the corresponding deficiency disease for most people. The other intake, which we consider to be the more important one, is the optimum intake, the one that leads to the best of health. For most vitamins this intake is much larger than the RDA and may be said to be in the megavitamin range.

There is now much information available about the optimum intake of vitamin C, but less about other vitamins and important nutrients. The problem of determining the values of the optimum intakes of nutrients, which is complicated by the phenomenon of biochemical individuality, is one of the most important public health problems today.

Despite this knowledge, many physicians are apt to tell you that large intakes of vitamin C and other vitamins have no value against cancer or any other disease and that these doses might themselves be so toxic as to result in death. A physician might say, for example, that a celebrated study at the Mayo Clinic has shown that vitamin C has no value in the treatment of patients with cancer. This conclusion is, however, wrong, as we show later in this book. Yet most physicians have been misled into believing that megavitamin treatment is a form of cancer quackery.

The sort of bias against vitamins that exists among most physicians and some biological scientists can be illustrated by the following statement in a report by a reviewer of an article by staff members in the Linus Pauling Institute of Science and Medicine: "When I began to read this article, I saw that the work had been done in the Linus Pauling Institute, and that accordingly it could not be accepted as reliable. Linus Pauling himself has been contending for years that megadoses of vitamin C have value in controlling the common cold and cancer, but these claims have been shown to be false." The statement that these claims have been shown to be false is, of course, not true, although many physicians still seem to accept it. The sort of logical error that has given rise to this position can be illustrated by the following anecdote. I was on a television program (the David Frost show) with one of the established "authorities" in nutrition, Dr Frederick Stare, then a professor at the Harvard School of Public Health. As the interview ended, Dr Stare said, "I know that Dr Pauling's method of preventing the common cold is no good because I tried it, and it didn't work." Before I could ask a question, David Frost said, "Gentlemen, I'm sorry that our time is up; I thank you for having been on the program." Then, after the TV camera had been turned off, Dr Stare turned to me and said, "Of course, I didn't use the astronomical amount that *you* recommend." Dr Stare has an M.D. degree but seems to have little knowledge of science and to be lacking in common sense. It takes only common sense to understand that the observation that a small dose of vitamin C did not stop a cold does not show that a megadose (an "astronomical" amount) would not be effective.

It may well be good that physicians find it difficult as individuals to accept a new idea in medicine, such as the use of large daily doses of vitamin C and other vitamins and minerals for the prevention and treatment of cancer. In the course of his training, a doctor is taught that he should apply to each patient the treatment that has been shown by experience probably to be the best for that patient, that is, for a patient with that disease. An outstanding specialist on diseases of the kidney, Dr Thomas Addis of Stanford Medical School (who died in 1949), has given an argument as to why doctors should not *think*, but should just follow the accepted practice in the treatment of a patient with a certain disease. Dr Addis himself had developed a new treatment for patients with chronic glomerular nephritis, a sort of kidney disease that was usually fatal. He had not been able to convince the medical establishment in general to accept his treatment. His effort to understand the situation led him through a rational argument to the conclusion that doctors should not think.

Here are his own words, in his book *Glomerular Nephritis*, published in 1948: "Quite properly, the actual treatment of patients is not usually the result of an explicit process of logical thought. In action the doctor should not have to find his way by a conscious process of inference. Whenever he is obliged to think, his purpose is endangered. For when he thinks, he will, like all other thinkers, surely make mistakes, and the errors, translated into action, may be disastrous. The patient trusts that his doctor knows, without thinking, what to do, and hopes that the prescription is not the outcome of the ratiocination of a single, fallible human being, but carries the signature of a great multitude of the scholars of disease and is validated by the accumulated experience of those who know and who do not need to think. So when we maintain that the theory of the treatment of glomerular nephritis involved the conscious exercise of thought, it is apparent that at this point we are leaving the realm of clinical tradition and practice and are entering the field of science and theory."

Granted, it is proper that the medical profession (and patients, too) should be cautious about new drugs. Drugs are dangerous. Almost all of them have seriously harmful side effects because of their toxicity, and sometimes these effects are not discovered until the drug has been given to thousands of patients. A cancer patient may have to try to balance the information given about the amount of benefit that a course of chemotherapy has provided to other patients with the same kind of cancer against the unpleasant and even dangerous side effects of the chemotherapeutic drug in deciding whether or not to accept the proposed therapy.

The extreme caution that should be followed with drugs does not, however, apply to orthomolecular substances, including the vitamins, which are characterized by their strikingly low incidence of toxic side effects. It is probably for this reason that it has been possible for many physicians to classify themselves as orthomolecular physicians, even though for the most part orthomolecular medicine has not been accepted by the medical establishment.

If we have not been able to convince physicians to recommend megavitamin therapy for cancer and other diseases, we have been somewhat more successful in making them understand that vitamins are not toxic. Many physicians, perhaps even a majority, have learned enough to be able to say to a patient, "So, you are taking very large amounts of vitamins; well, go ahead, if you want to – they may not help you, but they won't hurt you." This alone can give all of us hope for the future. If you have cancer, do not let your physician's statements prevent you from considering the possibility that megavitamins can help you. Do not give up hope.

– Linus Pauling

2 CLINICAL NUTRITION FOR TREATING AND PREVENTING CANCER

Anti-Cancer Vitamins and Minerals

No one can argue against the view that one has a better chance of dealing with a life-threatening disease if the general physical health is as good as is possible. One of the most important ways of achieving such a state of better health is to follow the principles of clinical nutrition, which we prefer to think is represented most fully by orthomolecular nutrition. Nutrients in optimum quantities improve the health of the individual. Because the main nutrients used in large doses are antioxidants, it is likely that they have anti-stress, anti-cancer, and anti-aging properties, and that they enhance the functioning of the immune system. Restoring good health and improving the immune system would improve one's chances against cancer, as it does against other diseases, but the nutrients have another role – they also enhance the efficacy of irradiation and chemotherapy, which like surgery are xenobiotic therapies since they are all foreign to the body, while at the same time decreasing their toxicity on the normal tissues of the body. Xenobiotic therapy aims to destroy or extirpate the lesion, but it also has many very toxic side effects, including the further suppression of the immune system. The optimum combination of orthomolecular therapy and xenobiotic therapy ought to improve the results of treating cancer substantially. What follows is a review of studies on the healing effects of vitamin C and other vitamins and minerals.

Vitamin C (Ascorbic Acid)

Although there was evidence in the medical literature that ascorbic acid used in optimum doses was therapeutic for cancer patients, it was not until Linus Pauling and Ewan Cameron published *Cancer and Vitamin C* in 1979 that there was a surge of interest in the scientific world, though the medical profession showed less enthusiasm for the subject. Several years earlier, Irwin Stone in *The Healing Factor: Vitamin C against Disease* concluded from his review of the enormous medical literature on this nutrient that vitamin C was helpful in the treatment of cancer. Higher vitamin C levels in animals were associated with a decrease in the incidence of cancer, and while most of the studies used small doses, Stone believed that much higher doses should be used, especially when vitamin C is one of the safest nutrients known. Stone cited one study that long before had suggested that low levels of vitamin C in the blood was a precondition for getting cancer. Supporting this view, A. Goth and I. Littmann found in 1948 that cancer started in organs whose ascorbic acid levels were under 4.5 mg per 100 mg. L. Benade, T. Howard and D. Burke, working in the laboratories of the National Cancer Institute, found that ascorbate was highly toxic to Ehrlich's ascites carcinoma and caused profound structural changes in the cancer cells; the Institute ignored this work, however.

Irwin Stone also recognized that many of the symptoms of leukemia were symptoms of scurvy. The white blood cells contained 20 to 30 times as much ascorbic acid as did normal cells. The huge volume of cells so rich in the vitamin sequestered the body's supply, producing scurvy in other tissues. He suggested that enough vitamin C be given to saturate these cells and leave enough for the rest of the body. He described the history of a man, 71 years old, with chronic myelogenous leukemia. After taking between 24.5 and 42 grams of vitamin C per day, he would not stop because he felt so much better. Twice, following his physician's orders, he stopped taking it, and in each case he developed fever and his spleen and liver became enlarged. These symptoms vanished 6 hours after resuming the vitamin. He died 18 months later from cardiac decompensation. At autopsy his spleen and liver were normal. His blood picture had not deteriorated while he was on the vitamin C.

In the 1990s, Ewan Cameron and his associates have provided more supporting data for the earlier Cameron and Pauling studies: their seminal discovery that megavitamin (large) doses of vitamin C prolonged life and improved its quality in Vale of Leven patients needs no review, as it is now firmly established in scientific and medical literature. In the past five years there has been much more interest in the connection between ascorbic acid and cancer as physicians have recognized that ascorbic acid is one of the most powerful natural antioxidants. Since free radical theories are sweeping the field, it now makes sense to consider all the natural antioxidants, of which vitamin C is one of the best known and most effective. B. Frei, L. England, and B.N. Ames report that ascorbate is the most effective water soluble antioxidant in human blood plasma, and suggest that it is a physiological antioxidant of major importance for protection against diseases and degenerative processes caused by oxidative stress. They even suggest that the RDA should be increased from 60 mg to 150 mg daily, thus pointing to the inadequacy of the present RDAs. M. Levine and associates have recommended that the optimum dose for young healthy men should be 300 mg per day, a five-fold increase over the RDA doses. The proceedings of a conference on "Antioxidant Vitamins and B-carotene in Disease Prevention," held in London, England, October 2-4, 1989, was published as a supplement to the *American Journal of Nutrition* in January 1991. The evidence showing the relationship between antioxidants such as vitamin C to cancer prevention and to other conditions was very powerful, leading Dr W.A. Pryor, who summed up the meeting, to conclude "that it may not be many years before the concept of the RDA is broadened, with one daily intake of a nutrient being recommended to prevent known vitamin deficiency diseases and a substantially higher value recommended to optimize the disease-preventing properties of these nutrients. Thus, there is reason for considerable hopefulness about our ability to reduce the incidences of the most life-limiting of the chronic diseases within the coming decades, with the consequent improvement in health, life span and well-being of our citizens."

Another important conference was held in Bethesda, Maryland, cosponsored by the National Cancer Institute, in September 1990. One of the factors leading to this meeting was Dr Pauling's persistent demand that the Institute examine seriously the claims that ascorbic acid was useful in the treatment of cancer. The main conclusions arising from this meeting supported the use of vitamin C for the treatment of cancer:

1. Ascorbic acid protects plasma lipids against oxidative damage. It scavenges free radicals, destroying them before they reach the membranes where they can do so much damage. In turn, uric acid protects ascorbic acid against destruction.

2. Ascorbic acid decreases the toxicity against normal tissue of drugs used in chemotherapy, and decreases the toxicity of radiation, but it did not protect the cancer. Thus, it increases the therapeutic index of both radiation and chemotherapy. One author recommended that it should always be given to patients who are given adriamycin. The degree of protection depended upon the dose. Low levels sufficient to protect against scurvy did not have any protective value against chemotherapy.

3. Ascorbic acid has anti-cancer properties. It protects cells against transformation into cancer by methylcholenthrene. It also protects avian cells against Rous sarcoma virus. Linus Pauling reported that ascorbic acid decreased the incidence and delayed the onset of malignant lesions (squamous cell carcinoma) in hairless mice exposed to ultraviolet. In another study it decreased the incidence of spontaneous mammary tumors in R 111 mice. Several other studies showed similar results.

4. An epidemiological survey of the field showed that in 33 out of 46 studies vitamin C was protective, decreasing incidence and mortality. Individuals in the top 25 percent had only 50 percent of the cancer risk of those in the lowest quarter.

5. Ascorbic acid has properties which make it an important part of any cancer treatment, and the stress-induced reduction of ascorbic acid by cancer therapy could be prevented or inhibited by the use of ascorbic acid.

In addition, H. Padh described some of the physiological and biochemical activities activated by ascorbic acid: it is required for collagen synthesis and stimulates the secretion of procollagen for the formation of extracellular matrix. Thus it can help to contain or to restrict the spread of cancer cells. It is needed for the biosynthesis of noradrenalin, for the activation of hormones. Its major role is to act as an antioxidant which minimizes damage caused by oxidative processes.

Ascorbic Acid Decreases Toxicity of Irradiation and Chemotherapy

Ascorbic acid has been proven to have yet another important role in the treatment of cancer. Vitamin C increases the killing effect (toxicity) of irradiation and of chemotherapy, and at the same time decreases the toxicity on normal tissue – i.e., it increases the therapeutic index. E. Cheraskin, W.M. Ringsdorf, and A. Brecher referred to an earlier study in which 54 women with cancer of the cervix were treated with irradiation. Half of the group were pre-treated for one week with a vitamin-mineral preparation containing vitamin C, and the other half were not. The treated group yielded the best response. K.N. Prasad and B.N. Rama reported the same effect. A.B. Hanck also concluded that ascorbic acid increased survival and decreased adverse effects of irradiation. In one study, after six months 67 percent of the vitamin treated group were free of symptoms, compared to 45 percent of the control group. Almost all listed side effects of irradiation were less frequent. Ascorbic acid reduces one of the dangerous side effects of chemotherapy and radiation, their mutagenic potential and poor tolerance.

Megadoses

The initial dose we used in our studies was 12 grams per day in three divided doses. Usually I advise patients to use the crystalline material rather than to swallow 24 of the 500 mg tablets. A few preferred to take the tablets. If they could tolerate this amount, they were advised to increase the dose slowly until it became almost like a laxative; it usually caused frequent bowel movements and gas when this sublaxative dose was exceeded. They would then decrease the dose to a value below this level with which they were comfortable. Most patients remained on at least 12 grams, but a few went much higher, up to 40 grams per day. After they were well for a few years, many of the patients would slowly decrease the dose to a level substantially below these levels. A few patients were also given intravenous ascorbic acid by their physicians. A very small number of patients could not tolerate even 50 mg of the ascorbic acid and could not follow the program. Today there is a vitamin C preparation called ester-C which is more tolerable for these very sensitive patients.

In 1972, Jay Patrick organized a world congress on vitamin C on the 50th anniversary of its discovery by Nobel Laureate Dr A. Szent Gyorgyi. Three other scientists were honored – Linus Pauling, Irwin Stone, and Fred Klenner. Dr Fred Klenner was the first physician to use ascorbic acid in large doses. He found it very effective in healing a large variety of diseases, whether given by mouth or given intravenously. At this meeting he described the response of a patient with breast cancer. She had a large mass in her breast and she had refused to take standard therapy. Instead, he gave her 100 grams of ascorbic acid intravenously daily. After several months, the tumor had stopped growing and was extruded by the normal breast tissue and the breast healed. Other orthomolecular oncologists are routinely using ascorbic acid in this way. At the 14th International Conference on Human Functioning, September 8-10, 1990, in Wichita, Kansas, Dr Riordan and his associates reported that by using cell cultures they were able to determine the amount of ascorbic acid that needed to be injected so that it would kill cancer cells. Used in these doses, ascorbic acid behaves like chemotherapy, but unlike all chemotherapy used routinely by oncologists, it has no toxicity – it does not kill normal cells. I have advised some of my cancer patients to use these large doses, up to 125 grams given over 4 to 6 hours without using the cell cultures assay.

During a recent international meeting of scientists interested in the possible relationship between vitamin C and cancer, two reports were presented which revealed a new way of considering the role played by vitamin C in maintaining health.

One study of a small series of healthy young men showed that increasing the daily intake of vitamin C to megadose levels did not increase the amount found in the blood in a straight line relationship. With increasing doses, the blood level of vitamin C increased after a few hours, but beyond that time, the level did not increase much. The fact that the increases in blood levels are limited has already created a feeling that megadoses are of no clinical value. The investigator nevertheless recommended that the daily intake ought to be at least 200 milligrams daily rather than the present RDA of about 50 milligrams.

Another study conducted by Dr Riordan focussed on the other end of the concentration scale as he studied why vitamin C reaches zero or crises levels in the blood. Dr Riordan had earlier reported that in *in vitro* cell culture studies, the toxicity of vitamins to certain cancer cell cultures did increase with increased amounts of this vitamin in the fluid. He reiterated Linus Pauling's explanation of how man and a few other animals lost the ability to make vitamin C many millions of years ago in the process of evolution, whereas most animals make their vitamin C on demand. While man must find vitamin C in his food or in supplements, most animals make it in their bodies by converting glucose into vitamin C. They make much more than we take in from our food; for example, a goat weighing about as much as a man will make 14 grams of vitamin C per day. These animals do not store large amounts but can make much more very quickly as demands increases. These demands are stress generated. Many years ago the decrease in the amount of vitamin C in rat adrenal glands was used as measure of the degree of stress and a vitamin C deficiency crisis level was determined.

As I see it, we need to consider not only the maximum levels of vitamin C which can be attained and sustained by high dose frequent dosing but also how to prevent the zero crises levels from occurring. It is possible that the incidence of cancer is more closely related to the number, frequency, and intensity of these crises than it is to the high doses than can be induced by oral supplementation. Dr Riordan's work points to this direction.

I asked Dr Riordan if he would prepare a brief summary of his work for this book. This is what he wrote:

"My odyssey of how I became interested in vitamin C as a therapeutic modality began in medical school. Because of a sore throat, I went to a very knowledgeable doctor who diagnosed a streptococcal infection. He offered me two options: he said aureomycin (the new antibiotic of the day) would clear up my problem in 3-4 days, or he said I could get rid of my streptococcal throat infection in a week by taking vitamin C. As a student living in near poverty, the choice between $7.00 for the aureomycin and 50 cents for the vitamin C was easy for me. I chose the vitamin C and all of my symptoms cleared within six days.

"Then in the late 1970s, I discovered something which amazed me. For many months, for research purposes, my plasma vitamin C was checked on a regular basis. It was always in the normal range, fluctuating between 1.3 to 1.7 mg percent, until the time I had a spider bite on my left thigh. The next morning I was scheduled for my periodic vitamin C level determination. The laboratory called me to report that no vitamin C was detectable. I thought, "Well, I'll fix that," and had one of our nurses give me 15 grams of vitamin C intravenously. To satisfy my curiosity and to determine the effectiveness of the intravenous vitamin C, the next morning I had my vitamin C rechecked. Again, to my amazement, no vitamin C was detectable. None was detectable each morning for the next four mornings, even though the previous day I would have had another 15,000 milligrams of vitamin C intravenously. Only on the fifth morning, when the bite was well on the way to resolution, did my plasma vitamin C begin to rise into the detectable 'scurvy' range. And it was several more days before my plasma reached its usual adequate vitamin C level.

"The spider bite episode led me to start measuring vitamin C in people on a regular basis. We studied sizeable groups like nurses before and after an eight hour shift, athletic teams during practice and before a game, and police rookies after an eight hour shift. These studies showed that it was apparently very easy to deplete one's vitamin C just by engaging in what for them was their usual work or activity. One police officer particularly stands out in my mind because at the end of night shift, both his urine and plasma had no detectable vitamin C. In addition to the stresses encountered by police officers, he had a rather deficient dietary intake during his shift. I vividly recall all he had during his busy eight hours were three cups of coffee, two cola drinks, and a chicken wing.

"Dr Mark Levine at the National Institutes of Health has made great strides in determining that normal people under normal circumstances require 200 milligrams of vitamin C daily, rather than the long recommended amount of 60 milligrams per day. Now, it is my hope that extensive studies to determine levels of vitamin C in response to factors such as stress, toxins, and insect bites will be forthcoming. At this point, we don't even know how much vitamin C is required to handle six mosquito bites.

"In one of my little books of vignettes of medical history, entitled 'Medical Maverick', I recount how physicians, as early as 1590, recognized the value of citrus fruits in preventing and treating scurvy. And, even though Dr John Woodall published in 1617 in *The Surgeons Notes* his advice of carrying lemon juice on voyages to prevent scurvy, more than a million sailors died of scurvy in the next 200 years. In 1753 Dr James Lind published his studies, performed on the crew of the *Salisbury*, demonstrating that citrus fruits effectively treated scurvy. His *Treatise on the Scurvy* went unnoticed and then went unheard. Forty years after Lind's death in 1794, his concept for the prevention of scurvy was finally put into practice.

"I can only hope that the scientific community will be moved to conduct studies to discover how much vitamin C humans need when experiencing crises of various kinds. In my opinion, that will lead to a totally different perception of how higher doses may benefit those who have had sudden reductions in their available vitamin C."

Dr Riordan's research suggests that we must place much more emphasis on preventing humans from reaching a crisis level of little or no vitamin C in their blood. Ideally, we would have a vitamin C infusion pump imbedded in us which would do for us what animals can do for themselves. Next best would be to take a dose of vitamin C every hour while awake. But hourly doses are not practical. Continuous intravenous infusion is practical and can readily be done in hospitals, a procedure that is already being examined. From this line of reasoning, all cancer cases should be given intravenous infusions for a matter of weeks or more at the beginning of their treatment for cancer.

Vitamin B-3 (Niacin or Niacinamide)

Vitamin C is not the only nutrient effective in treating and preventing cancer. Recent findings have shown that vitamin B-3 does have anti-cancer properties, most notably reported in 1987 at an international conference on "Niacin, Nutrition, ADP-Ribosylation and Cancer" in Texas, the eighth conference of this series. Niacin, niacinamide, and nicotinamide adenine dinucleotide (NAD) are interconvertable via a pyridine nucleotide cycle. NAD, the coenzyme, is hydrolyzed or split into niacinamide and adenosine dinucleotide phosphate (ADP-ribose). Niacinamide is converted into niacin, which in turn is once more built into NAD.

The enzyme which splits ADP is known as poly (ADP-ribose) polymerase, or poly (ADP) synthetase, or poly (ADP-ribose) transferase. Poly

(ADP-ribose) polymerase is activated when strands of deoxyribonucleic acid (DNA) are broken. The enzyme transfers NAD to the ADP-ribose polymer, binding it onto a number of proteins. The poly (ADP-ribose) activated by DNA breaks helps repair the breaks by unwinding the nucleosomal structure of damaged chromatids. It also may increase the activity of DNA ligase. This enzyme cuts damaged ends off strands of DNA and increases the cell's capacity to repair itself. Damage caused by any carcinogenic factor – radiation, chemicals – is thus to a degree neutralized or counteracted.

The 1987 Texas conference organizers have hypothesized that niacin prevents cancer. They treated two groups of human cells with carcinogens. The group given adequate niacin developed tumors at a rate only 10 percent of the rate in the group deficient in niacin. Dr M. Jacobson is quoted as saying, "We know that diet is a major risk factor, that diet has both beneficial and detrimental components. What we cannot assess at this point is the optimal amount of niacin in the diet. . . . The fact that we don't have pellagra does not mean we are getting enough niacin to confer resistance to cancer." About 20 mg per day of niacin will prevent pellagra in people who are not chronic pellagrins. The latter may require 25 times as much niacin to remain free of pellagra.

Vitamin B-3 may also increase the therapeutic efficacy of anti-cancer treatment. E. Kjellen and associates gave mice niacinamide, 0.2 g/kg body weight, 30 minutes before they were given radiation. One week earlier they had been injected with mammary adenocarcinoma cells. This is equivalent to 12 grams per day of niacinamide for an average human adult. The vitamin had no effect on tumor volume in these animals. However, the tumor volume decreased 86 percent after irradiation in niacinamide-treated mice, and remained 79 percent lower at four weeks. Mitotic activity remained low in niacinamide-treated animals after irradiation, but returned to pre-irradiation levels in non-treated mice. These authors suggested niacinamide may have a role in the treatment of malignant tumors.

In mice, niacinamide increased the toxicity of irradiation against tumors. In separate studies, M.R. Horsman, E. Kjellen, and I. Lee concluded that the combination of normobaric carbogen with nicotinamide could be an effective method of enhancing tumor radiosensitivity in clinical radiotherapy where hypoxia limits the outcome of treatment. D.J.

Chaplin and M.R. Horsman in independent studies found that nicotinamide was the best drug for increasing radiosensitivity compared to a series of analogues. This vitamin worked because it enhanced blood flow to the tumor. Nicotinamide also enhanced the effect of chemotherapy, according to a study by G. Chen and Q.C. Pan. Radiotherapy decreases the amount of nicotinamide adenine dinucleotide (NAD) in the liver by impairing the conversion of tryptophan to NAD, C. Streffer discovered. Both niacin and niacinamide are readily incorporated into NAD. Accordingly, it would be prudent for every patient receiving radiation to take supplemental vitamin B-3. This also applies to people exposed to irradiation from any source.

Other scientific studies have shown the efficacy of vitamin B-3 in treating and preventing cancer. H. Gotoh and associates have reported that nicotinamide significantly decreased urethane-induced malformations when given intraperitoneally to pregnant mice. A. Schmitt-Graff and M.E. Scheulen in two studies found that niacin decreased adriamycin cardiotoxicity in mice, but did not inhibit its antineoplastic activity, thus increasing its therapeutic index. They suggested that niacin may offer some cardioprotection during long-term adriamycin chemotherapy. Further evidence that vitamin B-3 is involved in cancer is the report by K. Nakagawa and associates that in animals there is a direct relationship between the activity of nicotinamide methyl transferase and the presence of cancer. Measuring the amount of N-methyl nicotinamide was used to measure the activity of the enzyme. In other words, in animals with cancer there is increased destruction of nicotinamide, thus making less available for the pyridine nucleotide cycle. This finding applied to all tumors except the solid tumors, Lewis lung carcinoma, and melanoma B-16.

Additional evidence that vitamin B-3 is therapeutic for cancer arises from the National Coronary Study conducted by P.L. Canner and associates. Between 1966 and 1975, five drugs used to lower cholesterol levels were compared to placebo in 8,341 men, ages 30 to 64, who had suffered a myocardial infarction at least three months before entering the study. About 6,000 were alive at the end of the study. Nine years later, only niacin had decreased the death rate significantly from all causes. Mortality decreased 11 percent and longevity increased by two years. The death rate from cancer was also decreased.

Vitamin E

Vitamin E includes the tocopherols of which d-alpha tocopherol succinate is the most active. It is the major lipid soluble antioxidant, protecting the polyunsaturated fatty acids in membranes against peroxidation. The usual intake is about 12 IU/d. Peroxidation of the pufa causes membrane damage. Vitamin E has other protective properties: it destroys nitrite which has been shown to increase the incidence of cancer; it protects the red blood cells in lungs against the toxic effect of ozone and hydroxyl radical toxicity. K.N. Prasad has reported that alpha tocopherol succinate induced differentiation in melanoma cells and inhibited the growth of neuroblastoma, rat glioma, and human prostate and melanoma cells induced by cAMP. K. Kline and R. Gopalakrishna also found it inhibited proliferation of human breast cells in culture.

Furthermore, G.W. Comstock and associates have shown that vitamin E has a weak protective effect against some of the cancers. More recent studies have shown in inverse relationship between levels of vitamin E in blood and the development of cancer. M.P. Longnecker and associates compared the vitamin E levels in 289 patients with cancer of the colon and rectum against 1267 matched controls. The E levels were slightly lower in the cancer cases. Similar findings were reported in studies led by by P. Knekt, P.R. Palan, and N. de Vries in the early 1990s. In another study led by P. Knekt, the alpha-tocopherol levels in 36,265 adults in Finland were studied. After eight years there were 766 cases of cancer. Persons with low levels had 1½ times the chance of getting cancer compared to the highest level. The association was strongest with gastrointestinal cancers and for other cancers not related to smoking. B.Y. LeGardeur and associates concluded from their data that lower vitamin E levels may be associated with lung cancer and to a greater degree than vitamin A, while A. Kornhauser and associates concluded that both beta carotene and vitamin E protect against the development of cancer and that they are chemopreventive.

The association between cancer and vitamin E consumption thus may not be strong, but an increasing number of reports appear showing that there is some connection. When so many variables are involved, it is very difficult to find very high correlations between the condition and the effect of only one of the nutrients. As long as we cannot be sure what are the most effective cancer preventive agents and therapeutic compounds, it seems only prudent to ensure that the subjects are obtaining enough vitamin E. The main question is how much is enough. As we have see with vitamin C and B-3, the role of the RDAs is being seriously questioned by many and recommendations have been made that for each disease there may be a unique RDA.

The Carotenoids

The role of carotenoids in preventing and treating cancer is a question for debate. One recent large scale Finnish study reported in the *New England Journal of Medicine* indicated that carotenoids may increase the incidence of lung cancer, and although the authors of the report hedged their conclusions with several reservations and qualifications, these were ignored by the daily press who frightened many patients with headlines such as those in the *New York Times* proclaiming "Vitamin Supplements Are Seen as No Guard Against Diseases" and "Study Sees No Benefit in Vitamins on Cancer or Heart Disease." This Finnish report on the effect of vitamin E and beta carotene on the incidence of cancer in male smokers is important, not because of its scientific value, but for the way it was treated in the national press. The news media headlines carried this grim message – vitamins may increase cancer – and this was the message that many of my patients received. For the next few days I received anxious calls, even though my patients are much more sophisticated about vitamins than are most individuals. They wanted reassurance that it was safe to continue with their vitamin C, vitamin E, and beta carotene. The media did not distinguish between the vitamins. There is a tendency in the public (including physicians) to have a global view of vitamins. If there is bad news about one, it means it is bad for them all. The vitamin critics were given one more opportunity to blast the use of vitamins – to return to their ancient position that only food was safe and no one needed vitamin supplements. But this is not what the dozens of authors of this study concluded. They found that these two antioxidants did not decrease the incidence of lung cancer, and because there was an increase in risk in the treated group, suggested the possibility that it might increase it.

Most studies, however, have shown the carotenoids to have anti-cancer effects. At a 1989 conference on "Antioxidant Vitamins and Beta Carotene in Disease Prevention" in London published as the proceedings in a

Supplement to the *American Journal of Clinical Nutrition*, Dr W.A. Pryor concluded, "At present, the strongest evidence for an anticarcinogen effect for the antioxidant nutrients appears to exist for beta carotene." Many other papers presented at the conference discussed the anti-cancer properties of beta carotene. The doses used ranged from 25,000 IU to 100,000 IU. The only hazard at the high doses is cosmetic.

Selenium

Although it is difficult to establish strong correlations between any one disease and any one nutrient when a large number of nutrient factors are involved, H.D. Foster in an excellent review concluded that the evidence for a negative correlation between selenium intake and the incidence of cancer was strong. In one 27-country survey, breast cancer mortality correlated strongly and negatively with dietary selenium (r = -0.80). Other minerals are also involved. A study of correlations coefficients in white males and soil levels in the United States showed that high soil selenium was negatively related to all cancer (-.52), positively correlated with very high soil mercury (0.59), and negatively correlated with very high soil calcium (-.47). However, case control studies yield conflicting data. Some workers find no difference in blood selenium levels between breast cancer and controls, while others find they are low in the cancer cases. Prospective studies also yield mixed data. One study on 4480 subjects, of whom 111 developed cancer, showed a significant but small decrease in selenium in the patients who developed cancer. More recent studies also give conflicting results.

While the anti-cancer effect of supplementing with selenium has not been examined extensively, there are some recent preliminary reports. S. Toma and associates measured selenium levels in 22 patients with precancerous lesions in the oral cavity, 10 with cancer and 13 controls. The selenium levels were 105, 77, and 101. They then administered selenium to the patients. In two patients, there was a complete remission, 5 showed a partial remission, 6 minor improvements, and with 5 there was no response. When the selenium was stopped, the growth resumed in 7 out of 18 cases. S. Yu and associates gave 300 micrograms of selenium in a double blind experiment to 40 healthy miners to test its safety. They concluded that this use of selenium was safe and effective to humans with low selenium status.

They found that selenium protected lymphocytes against DNA damage induced by ultraviolet radiation and the carcinogen 3,4 benzypyrene.

The frequent and recurring reports in the news media about the dangers inherent in excessive exposure to sunlight continually remind and frighten some people about the possibility of getting skin cancer. However, these reports do not discuss the connection between the nutritional health of the population and their susceptibility to cancer of the skin. Since ultraviolet radiation increases the formation of free radicals, it would not be surprising that increasing the availability of antioxidants would prevent some of the toxic reactions to ultraviolet radiation.

It has been shown that selenium is such a preventive nutrient. K.E. Burke and associates reported that selenium given to hairless pigmented mice protected them against damage from ultraviolet irradiation. They found that a lotion containing 0.02 percent L-selenomethionine or oral administration of water containing 1.2 ppm both were protective. These dosages did not cause any toxic reactions. They concluded that "SeMet is effective in protecting against skin cancer induced by UV irradiation, both by retarding the onset and reducing the number of lesions... [and] ...effective in reducing the acute damage induced by UV irradiation-inflammation (sunburn), blistering, and pigmentation (tanning)." No blisters developed in the treated mice during early weeks of irradiation, but they did develop in two-thirds of the control mice. They concluded with the practical suggestion that "protection might be provided by either topically or orally administered SeMet." In a subsequent report Burke confirmed these findings. She reported that both oral and topical selenium supplementation decreased the incidence and chronic damage from ultraviolet irradiation without being toxic. Mice treated with Se had a delayed onset and a markedly lesser incidence of skin cancer.

Selenium is a good antioxidant. It is synergistic with vitamin E, the body's best-known fat soluble antioxidant. The daily recommended dose is 200 micrograms. I have given 600 micrograms and more to certain patients for many years and have seen no toxic side effects. I would therefore suggest that the three best-known natural antioxidants – i.e., vitamin C, vitamin E, and selenium – be used to protect people against the toxic effect of excessive ultraviolet irradiation. The dose would be 200 micrograms selenium, 800 IU of vitamin E, and 3 or more grams per day of ascorbic acid. It should not take too much time to test these antioxidants in controlled studies. But because the danger from ultraviolet induced skin cancer and melanoma is potentially so great, it would appear to me to be prudent to take these simple nutrients as a precaution. They would, of course, have other advantages as well.

Selenium also has antidepressant properties. Using a double blind cross over design study, D. Benton and R. Cook gave 50 subjects 100 micrograms of selenium daily. They found that the lower the level of selenium in the diet the more frequent were reports of anxiety, depression, and fatigue following five weeks of selenium therapy. This mild antidepressant activity should be of value for all cancer patients.

Zinc and Copper

Zinc deficiency was not recognized over 30 years ago, but since then an association has been found with a large number of conditions such as growth retardation, skin disorders, delayed healing, birth defects, taste and smell disorders and loss of appetite, and immunological deficiency. Zinc deficiency induces immunodepression. Thymus-dependent acquired immunity is affected most severely. This is now well known and is becoming increasingly important because of the wide-spread inadequate intake of zinc. Zinc plays a large number of roles in host defense responses. Zinc contributes to plasma defense integrity and to functioning of binding sites. It inhibits phagocytic functions in high concentration. Low body stores of zinc are associated with dysfunction of T cells. Nucleic acid and protein synthesis is dependent on zinc. It plays a key role in metalloenzyme functions. From their review of the literature and their own research, C.C. Pfeiffer and M.R. Werbach in separate studies have suggested that this may explain some of the anticarcinogenic effects of zinc. In contrast, compounds which labilized lysosome enhanced tumor growth in animals. An increase in lipid peroxidation and labilization of lysosomes was inhibited, in CCl_4-induced liver injury, by zinc. With zinc deficiency, E.R. Tivers has shown that spleen and thymus decrease in weight, lymphocyte count is reduced, the response to antigens is decreased, immunoglobulin levels are decreased, T cell helper function is interfered with, and susceptibility to infection is increased. H.D. Foster examined the correlation coefficients between breast cancer and several soil constituents. For the years 1950 to

1967 in the United States there was a negative correlation between cancer incidence and very low zinc levels in soils. It was -0.52 with a 0.005 level of significance.

That zinc deficiency is related to cancer and that treatment with zinc may be therapeutic has been confirmed. There is also powerful evidence that the ratio of blood copper over blood zinc is a good measure of the presence and severity of the cancer. A.E. Bedrick and associates found copper and iron are present in melanoma, but not in nevi. Zinc was not present in either. Using toenail clippings, M.A. Rogers and associates found that zinc levels were lower in 379 cancer cases compared to 514 control subjects. Subjects at greatest risk for oral cancer had low zinc levels. Their selenium levels were also low.

In another extensive study led by S.K. Gupta, zinc copper values and their ratios were studied in 20 patients with benign breast disease, 35 with cancer, and 30 controls. They found the following values, suggesting that copper values and Cu/Zn ratios could be used as biochemical markers of cancer:

	Copper	Ratio Cu/Zn
Controls	99 ug/dl	0.86
Benign disease	118	0.86
Cancer	167	1.91

Similar findings were reported for cervical cancer by C.A. Chen and associates:

	Copper	Zinc	Ratio Cu/Zn
Controls	109	97	1.13
Stage 1	142		1.17
Stage 2	159		1.85
Stage 3 & 4	172	67	2.66

After surgery the values returned to normal.

D. Gal and associates used the marker level CA 125, greater than 35 ug/dl, copper levels higher than 150 ug/dl, and zinc less than 90 ug/dl as a panel for classifying patients with ovarian cancer. From their group, 32 were undergoing exploratory laparotomy, and 49 had definite ovarian cancer.

Most patients were Stage 3 and 4. The CA 125 serum level and a copper/zinc ratio over 1.65 provided the most sensitive panel for diagnosing ovarian cancer before operation. In 14 out of 14 who had cancer the panel was correct in predicting cancer, while in 13 out of 14 with no clinical evidence for cancer the panel was correct in predicting cancer was not present. Second-look operations could have been replaced by this diagnostic panel. H.F. Goode and associates found zinc plasma levels lowest in patients with gastrointestinal cancer and polymorphonuclear cells. Similar findings were made for cancer of the head, neck, and face by G.B. Toke and B.K. Dhamne. Alterations in copper/zinc values and their ratios were related to the stage of the disease. These authors suggested that Cu/Zn ratios could be used to diagnose and to monitor treatment. The ratio was more reliable than the individual values.

Similar findings were made by S.L. Lian and associates. Copper/zinc ratios were elevated in patients with nasophryngeal carcinoma, more so in the later stages. Essentially similar findings have been reported in studies led by M. Diez, N. Cetinkaya, M. Ebadi, T. Hisake. Diez found that a value of 1.72 of copper/zinc discriminated between cancer patients and healthy controls with a sensitivity of 89 percent, positive predictive value of 92 percent, specificity of 84 percent and negative predictive value of 92 percent. The ratio also was predictive of prognosis. Patients with ratios over 2.25 had less than 5 percent survival over two years, while patients with ratios under 1.72 had a 70 percent survival expectancy. These authors found this ratio more sensitive in diagnosing lung cancer than chest radiographs, sputum cytologic studies, bronchoscopic brachial washings, and plasma carcinoembryonic antigen levels. There was only one intervention study of zinc and copper abstracted in the past five years. J. Wahrendorf and associates supplemented the diet of people living in a high risk area in China for esophageal cancer. They found that individuals who showed large increases in retinol, riboflavin, and zinc blood levels were more likely to have histologically normal esophagus at the end of the trial.

It is possible that the high copper/zinc ratios in cancer patients are caused by the increased level of copper in blood which may be an attempt by the body to control cancer growth. Copper increases the formation of free radicals and these are used by leucocytes to kill cancer cells. Copper and iron increase the oxidation of catechol amines to their chrome indoles like adrenochrome. Adrenchrome is an anti mitotic, an anti-cancer compound. There is an inverse relationship between copper and zinc. A deficiency of one will cause an increase in the amount of the other. The easiest way to bring down copper levels is to increase the intake of zinc. Fortunately, zinc is a very safe trace mineral and can be given in useful dosages for long periods of time with hardly any side effects.

In summary, patients with cancer have elevated serum copper levels, elevated ratios of copper/zinc, and may have low zinc levels. The higher the ratios are, the more malignant is the disease and the poorer the prognosis. It is likely that these indices will become generally used in helping with the diagnosis, in following treatment, and in estimating prognosis.

With all this evidence of the importance of zinc, I decided to include adequate zinc in the supplemental program for the cancer patients who came to me for nutritional advice. I used the following compounds: zinc sulfate 220 mg, zinc gluconate 50 mg, and zinc citrate 50 mg daily.

Antioxidants Used in Combination

As early as 1945 Dr M. Gerson treated a series of cancer patients with special diets and with some nutrients, including niacin 50 mg 8 to 10 times per day, dicalcium phosphate with vitamin D, vitamins A and D, and liver injections. He found that all the cancer cases were benefitted in that they became healthier, and in many cases the tumors regressed. In a subsequent report, Gerson elaborated on his diet: he now emphasized a high potassium over sodium diet, ascorbic acid, niacin, brewer's yeast, and lugol's iodine. Right after the war there was no ready supply of vitamins as there is today. I would consider the use of these nutrients in combination very original and enterprising. Dr Gerson was the first physician to emphasize the use of multivitamins and some multiminerals.

Other multi-antioxidant nutrient studies are beginning to appear. K.E. Brock and associates have found that high plasma beta carotene levels reduced the risk of developing cervical cancer by 80 percent, high ascorbic acid in addition reduced it to 60 percent, and increased consumption of fruit juice to 50 percent. Fruit juice contains bioflavonoids, also antioxidants. G. McKeown-Eyssen and associates found a slight reduction in risk using small, inadequate doses of vitamin C 400 mg and vitamin E 400 mg. In a study led by V. Noto, either vitamin C or E inhibited the growth of breast carcinoma, epidermoid carcinoma, and endometrial adenocarcinoma in vitro, but when both were combined, there was a pronounced synergistic effect. Ten to 50 times lower concentrations were as effective. The inflicted damage was dramatic and irreversible. Other studies led by G.I. Kallistratos and R.J. Winn agree upon the anti-cancer effect of the use of multinutrients. A multivitamin megadose study on bladder cancer led by L.M. Lamm showed a significant improvement over the use of RDA doses when measured by recurrences and by longevity. The five year estimate of recurrences was 91 percent with RDA doses and 41 percent in the megadose group. The first group survived 18.6 months and the megadose group 33 months, but because of the small number of patients per group, this was not statistically significant. The study group used adequate doses of vitamin A, pyridoxine, vitamin D-3, vitamin E, and zinc, but, in my opinion, inadequate amounts of vitamin C and the other B-vitamins. Yet their results were very significant. In another study, Lamm and associates found that their patients after surgery had a much better prognosis when treated with megadose vitamin therapy. The only vitamins they used in megadose levels were vitamin A 40,000 IU, vitamin B-6 100 mg, vitamin C 2,000 mg, vitamin E 400 IU, and zinc 90 mg. The control group received only RDA doses. The recurrence rate over 5 years was 80 percent out of 30 patients in the control group and only 40 percent out of 35 patients in the megavitamin group ($P< 0.0011$).

In the conclusion to his study of the efficacy of multinutrients, using a multinutrient program very similar to the orthomolecular regimen used in our studies, Dr Rueff concluded, "It is evident that these effects are positive. The following results are noted: better tolerance to chemotherapy and/or radiotherapy with lessened fatigue and mental depression, better preservation of immune and medullary functions, general and psychic state, skin and hair, adjuvent effect against nausea, vomiting and diarrhea. We never observed toxic or negative effects with these doses. On the contrary, it always seems that the overall result in quality and duration of life is better. The best evidence is that the patients themselves demand these supplements."

The ideal cancer chemoprevention would be food which contained all the natural antioxidants in the optimum amounts. However, such an ideal diet is not available. During evolution we have come to use what is present in food, not simply one antioxidant at a time. Since we do not have such an ideal diet, the next best preventative and therapeutic regimen is to use as many antioxidants as we can in combination with the best food available. This we call the orthomolecular regimen.

– Abram Hoffer

The Orthomolecular Regimen

There is clearly good evidence that the regular ingestion of mega amounts of vitamin C (1 to 20 grams per day) and of other vitamins increase the state of health and well-being, increase the length of life, and decrease the incidence of cancer, heart disease, diabetes, and other diseases. Much of this evidence is discussed in our previous books, notably *How To Live Longer and Feel Better* and *Hoffer's Laws of Natural Nutrition*. We estimate that this prophylactic effect, together with the therapeutic regimen described in the present study (used for cancer and also for other disease), would increase life expectancy for those who follow the orthomolecular lifestyle by an average of 24 years. If you should become ill with cancer, heart disease, or other serious disease, you should begin the therapeutic orthomolecular regimen immediately, as an adjunct to appropriate conventional therapy.

The main kinds of conventional therapy for cancer are surgery, high-energy radiation, and chemotherapy. Surgery can be recommended when the size and location of the malignant growth are such that its complete surgical removal is feasible; surgery then often leads to a cure. The orthomolecular regimen should be begun before surgery and continued steadily in order to facilitate healing and to potentiate the immune system, so as to prevent the formation of metastases by migrant malignant cells released into the circulation and to control infections. Of the 134 patients in our study, 61 percent had received surgery before being entered into the study and 10 afterward. Surgery is a possibility for almost all kinds of cancer.

Radiotherapy (treatment with high-energy radiation, usually high voltage x-ray or gamma rays, sometimes neutrons or protons), is often used together with surgery in the effort to destroy remaining malignant cells. When used alone, radiotherapy is often effective against some cancers, including skin cancers and deeply invasive cancers of the bladder. A disadvantage is that these rays are toxic not only to the malignant cells but also to the normal cells, so that the patient suffers from nausea and other side effects. These side effects can be controlled, however, by the massive intake of vitamin C. For this reason and others it is wise not to stop the orthomolecular regimen during the period of irradiation. Of the patients in this study 40 percent received radiotherapy before entry into the study and 16 percent afterward.

Chemotherapy, the use of drugs such as 5-fluorouracil and methotrexate (there are many others) that are toxic to malignant cells (and also to normal cells), was given to 32 percent of the patients before entry into this study and 17 percent afterward. The fraction of patients with advanced ('untreatable') cancer who receive chemotherapy varies widely from country to country. In Europe this fraction is less than 10 percent, in Canada (for example, in this study) about 40 percent, and in the United States about 80 percent. This kind of treatment, sometimes with several different chemotherapeutic drugs, has very limited value for most kinds of cancer, but is by itself effective against leukemias and related malignancies of the lymphoid system. Chemotherapy, like radiotherapy, has the disadvantage that it causes disagreeable side effects. These side effects are, however, largely suppressed by a high intake of vitamin C. It is accordingly important for the patient to continue following the orthomolecular regimen throughout the course of the chemotherapy.

A statement that we have made repeatedly is that we strongly recommend the orthomolecular regimen to all cancer patients as an adjunct to appropriate conventional therapy. An important word in this statement is the adjective 'appropriate'. If there is good evidence that the proposed conventional therapy has been found to be sufficiently effective in the treatment of other patients with the same kind of cancer to outbalance the disagreeable side effects of the treatment, then the patient should give serious consideration to the possibility of accepting the treatment, but if there is no such evidence, then the patient should reject the proposed therapy. Dr Ewan Cameron has said that in Scotland the physicians follow the policy that a kind of therapy should not be used unless there is evidence that its probable benefit is greater than the harm it does, and accordingly chemotherapy is used only for patients for whom an overall benefit from its use would be expected. A patient for whom there is no longer hope for a curative conventional therapy or a palliative conventional therapy is given good nursing care, with administration of opiates as needed to control pain, and is not subjected to the inconvenience and misery of some treatment, or, in some hospitals, is treated with vitamin C or other orthomolecular regimen. In the United States, however, and to some extent in Canada, the policy that is followed seems to be that some treatment should continue to be administered in order that the patient not lose hope. This attitude is illustrated by the statement of one physician to another, "Yes, the chemotherapy was successful: it gave the patient the delusion that the disease was being treated."

Cancer of the colon and rectum can serve as an example. There is rather general agreement that with this kind of cancer the most that can be expected of treatment with chemotherapeutic drugs is some retardation of the growth of the malignant tumor, but this response is highly predictable and the side effects are so disagreeable as to make the value of the treatment doubtful. In 1978 Dr Charles G. Moertel, a prominent investigator of cancer therapies, stated, "There is no solid evidence that treatment with fluorinated pyrimidines contributes to the overall survival of patients with gastrointestinal cancer regardless of the stage of the disease at which they are applied," and in 1985 he and his associates wrote, "We felt ethically justified in studying this group of patients without first offering cytotoxic drugs because in our opinion there is no known form of chemotherapy for colorectal cancer that has been demonstrated to produce substantive palliative benefit or extension of survival." Nevertheless, before their study of 101 patients with advanced colorectal cancer was ended, they had administered 5-fluorouracil or some other chemotherapeutic drug to 58 of these patients. An analysis of the reported survival times of these patients showed that the chemotherapy had in fact *shortened* their lives.

We may ask why Dr Moertel and his associates could have decided to give chemotherapy to their patients after having stated that it has no value. An answer to this question was given by Dr Moertel himself, who said that it is important to continue the treatment: "Patients with advanced gastrointestinal cancer and their families have a compelling need for a basis of hope. If such hope is not offered, they will quickly seek it from the hands of quacks and charlatans."

We are convinced that the nutritional regimen described in this book, used together with appropriate conventional therapy, has significant value for every patient with cancer, and we recommend that it be initiated as early as possible in the course of the disease. Moreover, the use of dietary supplements by people in ordinary health, together with other health practices, can decrease the incidence not only of cancer, but also of heart disease and other diseases and slow down the process of aging.

– Linus Pauling

Every patient in the series discussed in this book had already, before entry into our study, been diagnosed as having cancer, and all but 14 from the original series of 134 had received one or more of the usual treatments – surgery, high-energy radiation, and chemotherapy – with 30 having received all three. Most had either failed to respond or were suffering a relapse at the time of entry; a few were well but hoped that they could find a treatment that would keep them healthy. They all knew a fair amount about cancer and their chances of surviving their disease. They were depressed, anxious, angry, and upset, but almost all of them were hopeful and determined to survive. They frequently needed their determination to persuade the family doctor to make the referral, especially early in this study. Several had made plans to visit clinics in Mexico, but were instead diverted to see me.

Several topics were discussed during the first interview. Whenever a family member or friend came with the patient, he or she was invited into my office, with the patient's approval. Spouses invariably wanted their mates to be there. The subjects discussed by me were (1) hope, (2) faith, (3) visualization, (4) the need to live, (5) food, (6) nutritional supplements, and (7) drugs for psychiatric problems. These topics were not necessarily discussed in this order and some were not discussed with patients already familiar with these factors in cancer therapy.

Hope and faith are essential, for without hope or faith a patient would not follow any treatment. There must be enough to motivate the patient to follow what is at first a complicated program. Hope is an essential component of every therapeutic relationship. In my opinion, the expression "false hope" has no meaning; either there is hope or there is no hope. A patient with no hope will not try, and certainly would not have been in this study unless severely depressed or anxious. A patient placed in a dying role will no longer expect treatment for cancer to be useful, but may want relief from depression and anxiety as well as from pain. Many of these patients have been deprived of hope by their oncologists when they were told that nothing more could be done or that there was no treatment for their cancer – even before they were treated. For example, one patient, after her laparotomy and bypass operation, was told that she would be dead in three months and that she should immediately write her will. She was alive and well 18 years later in 1996.

The advice given to the patient about foods includes increasing the intake of fruits and vegetables and decreasing that of meat. Also the intake of sugar should be severely reduced. A good amount of water should be ingested every day, but not in the form of soft drinks, which contain either sugar or artificial sweeteners, which might be harmful.

The most important part of the regimen is the dietary supplements. Vitamin C (ascorbic acid, sodium ascorbate) may be the most important for controlling cancer, but there is good evidence that the other vitamins are also important, perhaps equally important, and that some minerals, especially zinc and selenium, also have value. It can be seen from the case histories recorded in this book that most of the supplements were taken by mouth in divided doses three times a day, usually after meals, with some, for convenience, taken only once a day.

In this study vitamin C was given orally in amounts from 3 to 40 grams per day, usually 12 grams. This might be taken as four 1,000 mg tablets after each meal. An alternative is to take this vitamin as pure crystalline ascorbic acid or sodium ascorbate or the 50-50 mixture of the two. One level teaspoonful is about 4 grams. The crystals can be dissolved in water, orange juice, or some other fruit juice. Ascorbic acid in water is rather sour, but less sour in fruit juice, which buffers the acid. Sodium ascorbate is almost tasteless, and the 50-50 mixture is pleasantly acidic. The pure crystals in 1-kilogram jars are the cheapest form of vitamin C.

Vitamin C is a laxative. A very large intake may cause too much looseness of the bowels. A cancer patient may obtain the best protection by taking a daily amount a little less than the bowel-tolerance limit, which for the seriously ill patient may be quite high, such as 60 grams per day (four level tablespoons of the crystals). The limit decreases as control over the cancer is achieved.

Some patients in this study were also given sodium ascorbate by intravenous infusion. Dr Cameron's patients in Vale of Leven Hospital in Scotland were all given between 10 and 40 grams per day for two weeks by intravenous infusion, as well as 10 grams daily orally, continued indefinitely. As much as 150 grams has been administered by intravenous infusion in one day, with good response.

Vitamin B-3, either niacin or niacinamide, was also given to the patients in this study. The daily intake was either 1.5 grams or 3 grams (a 500 mg tablet or two tablets three times per day). Niacin is rejected by some patients because of the flushing reaction (tingling of the skin), but this reaction usually stops after a few days. Niacinamide, which probably is nearly as effective against cancer, does not cause this reaction.

Many of the patients in this study were also given vitamin E, usually one 800 IU capsule per day. We recommend either this amount or twice as much to all cancer patients. Vitamin E (tocopherol) is not a simple substance. There are several tocopherols, differing somewhat in their biological activity, so that 800 IU may be contained in a small capsule or require a larger one. We do not know that one tocopherol is more effective than another in controlling cancer; hence we recommend the cheapest one (per IU). Recent cell culture studies suggest d-alpha tocopherol succinate may be more effective than the other forms.

It is likely that an increased intake of all of the B vitamins is helpful in controlling cancer. Part of the evidence is that several epidemiological studies have shown that a high intake of vegetables that contain the B vitamins in good amounts is correlated with a decrease in incidence of several kinds of cancer. In the present study the B vitamins were at first not

TABLE 3

Composition of a Super B Tablet (from Bronson Pharmaceuticals)

B-1	50 mg
B-2	50 mg
B-3 (niacinamide)	50 mg
B-6	50 mg
B-12	0.100 mg
folic acid	0.400 mg
biotin	0.400 mg
pantothenic acid	100 mg

included in the regimen (except B-3) or were included in an ordinary B-complex tablet per day, containing just the usually recommended small amounts, the RDAs. Later patients received one tablet per day containing as much as 100 times the RDAs of several of the B-vitamins. Those tablets may be called Super B, B-50, or B-100. The composition of Super B, for example is given in Tables 3, 4 and 5. The total weight of these vitamins is only half a gram, so that only one tablet is needed.

Twelve tablets each day of this preparation will provide almost the entire program that I have been using over the past five years for cancer treatment. It will provide daily 12 grams of vitamin C as ascorbates, 120 mg of vitamin B-3, 60 mg of vitamin B-6, 300 IU of vitamin E, 30,000 IU of beta carotene, 600 micrograms of selenium, 60 mg of zinc plus the other nutrients. The only addition needed would be more vitamin B-3 and more beta carotene for some individuals.

TABLE 4
Composition of a Supergram C Tablet (from Alacer Corporation)
(Each two tablets contains the following amounts)

Vitamin C as mineral ascorbates (as salts of calcium, magnesium, potassium, zinc, and chromium)	2000 mg
8 mixed bioflavonoids	25 mg
quercitin	25 mg
thiamine	15 mg
riboflavin	17 mg
vitamin B-3	20 mg
pyridoxine	10 mg
B-12	6 mcg
vitamin E, mixed tocopherols	15 I.U.
pantothenic acid	10 mg
d-biotin	300 mcg
folic acid	400 mcg
beta carotene	5000 I.U.
selenium	100 mcg
iodine	25 mcg
calcium, as ascorbate	70 mg
magnesium, as ascorbate	70 mg
zinc, as ascorbate	10 mg
manganese, as ascorbate	2 mg
molybdenum, as ascorbate	1 mg
chromium, as ascorbate	100 mcg

TABLE 5
Composition of 12 capsules (Daily Intake) of the Ruth Harrell Vitamin Mineral Capsules (from Bronson Pharmaceuticals)

vitamin A (palmitate)	15,300 I.U.
vitamin D (cholecalciferol)	300 I.U.
thiamine mononitrate (B-1)	300 mg
riboflavin (B-2)	200 mg
niacinamide (B-3)	750 mg
calcium pantothenate	490 mg
pyridoxine hydrochloride(B-6)	350 mg
cobalamin (B-12)	0.100 mg
folic acid	0.400 mg
vitamin C (ascorbic acid)	1500 mg
vitamin E (D-a-tocopheryl) succinate	600 I.U.
magnesium (oxide)	300 mg
calcium (carbonate)	400 mg
zinc (oxide)	30 mg
manganese (gluconate)	3 mg
copper (gluconate)	1.75 mg
iron (ferrous fumarate)	7.5 mg
calcium phosphate ($CaHPO_4$)	37.5 mg
iodide (KI)	0.15 mg

Many of the patients were also given vitamin A, 10,000 to 50,000 IU per day, and its precursor, beta carotene, 10 to 75,000 units per day, or both. We recommend that these substances be taken.

Among the minerals, many patients received zinc 50 to 220 mg per day, selenium 0.200 to 0.600 mg per day, and some also received compounds of magnesium and calcium. These supplementary minerals, and also other minerals in the usual amounts, may well have value for patients with cancer.

It is not necessary to take a separate tablet or capsule for each vitamin and mineral. For example, by checking the catalogs of mail-order retailers of vitamins, one can find products that provide most of the desired nutrients, as recommended above, in a single formulation, which may then be supplemented by two or three others to make up the deficit. Care must be taken to check the prices so as not to waste money by buying high-priced vitamins that are claimed to more effective than other brands.

Another preparation of vitamin-mineral capsules from Bronson

Pharmaceuticals used by Dr Ruth Harrell and her associates in treating cancer is also recommended. Twelve of these capsules per day would come close to providing the nutrients used in the present study, needing to be supplemented by a large amount of vitamin C, a gram or two of niacin or niacinamide, around 0.5 mg of selenium, and 100 to 200 mg of zinc.

It is our opinion that every patient with cancer should follow this regimen for the rest of their lives, without missing a day. People who do not have cancer or never have had cancer may follow a similar regimen to improve their general health, to decrease the incidence of cancer, heart disease, and other disease, and to slow down the process of aging. For these prophylactic purposes, an intake of vitamins and minerals one half to one quarter as great as recommended for cancer patients may suffice.

– Abram Hoffer

3

CLINICAL STUDIES OF THE VALUE OF ORTHOMOLECULAR TREATMENT

Clinical Methodology

About 1952, a woman was admitted to the psychiatric ward of the General Hospital in Regina, Saskatchewan, where I was starting our research program in psychiatry. After surgery for breast cancer, the irradiated area of her breast had become infected and ulcerated; she had also developed a psychosis her psychiatrist believed could be best treated with electroconvulsive therapy (ECT). For reasons I have now forgotten, I asked her psychiatrist to withhold treatment, as I wanted to investigate the effect of ascorbic acid on her psychosis. The dose would be 3 grams per day (1 g t.i.d., 3 times each day). Her psychiatrist agreed to delay ECT for three days, though I had hoped to have several weeks. Thus I decided to give her much more ascorbic acid than I usually prescribed for my patients. I started her on ascorbic acid 1 gram each hour. If she slept for four hours, she would be given the 4 grams she had missed. The vitamin was started on a Saturday morning. By the following Monday morning she had received 45 grams. To everyone's surprise, she was mentally normal. The psychiatrist cancelled the ECT and she was discharged a few days later. We also observed that the ulcerated lesion had begun to heal for the first time. It did not occur to me that the ascorbic acid might have value in treating her cancer, so preoccupied was I with psychiatry. She lived another six months, free of psychosis. She was not given any follow-up ascorbic acid.

In 1960 I started to examine urine from schizophrenic patients for the presence of a substance rarely found in non-schizophrenic subjects. We first found it in the urine of alcoholic patients given 200 micrograms of D-lysergic acid diethylamide (LSD). The substance developed a mauve color on the paper chromatogram which had not been present before the patient was given the LSD. We began to examine the effect of LSD following the hypothesis that, inasmuch as LSD caused a schizophrenic-like state in non-schizophrenic subjects, a similar substance might be causing similar biochemical changes in the schizophrenic patients. If we could find something in the urine after the administration of LSD that was not normally present, we could then compare schizophrenic patients with controls. A large number of patients and non-patients were examined.

We called the substance the mauve factor. Later it was identified as kryptopyrrole (KP). It was found most frequently in early schizophrenic patients before they were treated and was not present when they recovered, no matter how they were treated. To rule out stress, we examined many seriously sick patients from the medical and surgical wards. KP was found more commonly in patients with cancer of the lung. Out of 299 physically ill patients, 12 percent excreted KP, but from 146 cancer patients, 30 percent excreted it, including seven out of eight patients with lung cancer. In every psychiatric case no more was excreted after treatment. I did not examine the urine of cancer patients after treatment.

In 1977 a woman with obstructive jaundice was found at laparotomy to have an inoperable cancer of the head of the pancreas. She was given a bypass and advised she had only a few months to live. A few weeks later she was referred to me. She had started to take ascorbic acid 10 grams daily. She had read Norman Cousins's book *The Anatomy of an Illness* (1979), and when she told her physician, he advised her to see me. I increased her dose to 40 grams and added other nutrients. By that time I had been using multiple nutrients for the patients who were referred to me. Six months later her tumor was gone. She is still alive and well today. One case does not constitute proof, but like the white crow, it suggests that there is something there worth looking into.

I then recalled two earlier patients, the first a retired professor who developed inoperable bronchiogenic cancer of the lung. The biopsy was positive and the tumor was visualized by bronchoscopy. While he was being investigated, he became psychotic (depression and personality change). It was assumed that he had metastases to his brain, which made the lesion inoperable; he was instead treated by irradiation. When the radiation series was completed, he was confused and disoriented, with visual and auditory hallucinations. He was also delusional and irrational, and his memory and power of concentration were impaired. Not surprisingly, he remained depressed. His diagnosis was organic confusional psychosis, probably due to secondaries from his lung cancer. Five months later he was discharged to his home. His wife and a special nurse's aide as an assistant were not able to cope with him, and he was re-admitted two weeks later to our psychiatric ward, worse than he had been. Terminal care was authorized and he was to be held until a place could be found where he could die. Following this last admission, I had his urine tested. He excreted huge quantities of KP, so much that the area on the paper chromatogram was blood red, not mauve.

I suggested to his treating psychiatrist that he start him on niacin 1 g t.i.d. and ascorbic acid 1 g t.i.d. By then we had completed several double-blind controlled clinical experiments that showed that schizophrenic patients given these vitamins had a much higher recovery rate than those given a placebo. Non-blind clinical studies showed that any patient excreting KP, no matter what the diagnosis, responded much better to these vitamins than to no treatment. The presence of KP was an indication for using these vitamins. After three days, this patient was mentally normal. He could not remember anything that had happened over the months of psychosis, though he knew about his cancer and his terminal prognosis. I believed he would need maintenance vitamins, and he agreed to remain on the program. After discharge he came to see me each month to pick up a fresh supply of vitamins. To my surprise, he remained well for 30 months, and after 12 months his chest x-ray was clear. The head of the cancer clinic told me that with each three months of follow-up the shadow became less prominent until it was gone. When he eventually died at age 76, an autopsy was not done, but he did not die from his cancer.

I saw the second case about a year later. I advised a 16-year-old girl with Ewings sarcoma of the right arm to take niacinamide 3 grams and ascorbic acid 3 grams daily. She was booked for surgery to amputate her arm, but her surgeon was persuaded to wait for a month. She made a complete recovery and is still well 35 years later. I concluded that the main therapeutic factor was the vitamin B-3 (niacin or niacinamide) as it is for schizophrenia. It does have anti-tumor properties. After studying Ewan Cameron and Linus Pauling's *Cancer and Vitamin C*, I was convinced, however, that the main therapeutic nutrient was vitamin C and that vitamin B-3 had lesser anti-tumor properties.

I became determined to pursue these leads more seriously in 1978, following the death of my sister from breast cancer and the death of my father from prostate cancer. After I moved my practice from Regina to Victoria, British Columbia, the first patient with cancer I saw recovered on vitamin therapy. She was so grateful she began to tell her relatives and friends about her recovery. Ironically, the only one who did not believe her was her younger brother, a psychiatrist, who "knew" vitamins could not help anyone. Gradually more cancer patients were referred to me. The increase in the number of referrals was steady. In the three years 1976-1979 there were 3, in 1981 there were 6, in 1984, 12, in 1986, 12, and in 1988, 50, a total of 134.

The increase in referrals was the result of increasing familiarity with nutrition and nutrients by patients living in British Columbia and by their physicians. As physicians saw what was happening to their cancer patients who had been referred to me, they became more willing to refer others. Over a period of four years, the marked shift in attitude of national cancer societies from rejection to cautious acceptance of the role of nutrition in cancer must have made it easier for these referrals to be made.

It is difficult for physicians to refer cancer patients to a psychiatrist unless there are also psychiatric problems. However, patients who are told they have cancer and especially patients who are dying from cancer do have psychiatric problems, even though they are not primarily mentally ill.

In 1985 after I had seen 41 patients, I realized that the patients given at least 12 grams of ascorbic acid daily had a better outlook. For patients seen between 1978 and 1983, out of 11 who did not follow the nutrient regimen, none were alive and the mean survival was 4.8 months, while out of 26 who took the full dose of vitamin C, 18 were alive, for a mean survival of 16.2 months.

With prompting from Dr Pauling, I began a follow-up study of every patient I had treated from 1978-1988 to determine their outcome. I sent this data to Dr Pauling for his analysis. In the first study, 134 patients seen between August 1977 and March 1988 were followed until 31 December 1989. We concluded that orthomolecular treatment given to female related cancers had improved life expectancy about 20 times compared to our non-random controls and 12 times for other cancers. In our second paper, a second cohort of 170 patients seen from April 1988 to 31 December 1989 was followed to 31 December 1992. These results were about the same as those we had earlier published. We concluded that while vitamin C alone led to about 10 percent excellent responders, the addition of the other nutrients increased this to about 40 percent.

For a 1992 conference in Tulsa, I examined the first cohort of 134 further. In the first year after treatment, 75 percent of the control group of 33 died compared to 25 percent from the treated group of 101. On 1 January 1992, 41 patients were still alive from the treated group and one from the control. The average survival was 49 months for the treated group compared to 15 months for the control. The survival data suggested that the original Hoffer and Pauling estimates of survival were not far off the mark. As of 31 December 1993, 34 were still alive from the treated group and none from the controls. By 1 July 1996, 33 were alive, 24 having lived 10 years, 4 died, and 7 will probably live 10 years. The 10-year survival will probably be about 30 percent out of the original group of 101.

Double Blind vs Cohort Controlled Studies

In this study the main vitamin was ascorbic acid, but I also used vitamin B-3, either niacin or niacinamide, as well as other nutrients. This approach may be criticized by some, especially those who are convinced that only a prospective double-blind controlled study can be scientific. Ethically, it was impossible for me to withhold from any patient whatever treatment that might improve the chance of controlling his or her cancer. In each case, the two of us, my patient and I, worked together to treat the disease. If I had had to withhold, for example, vitamin B-3 just to satisfy those who believe in testing only one substance per study, I could not in good conscience have continued to treat my patient, knowing or believing that I was not doing my best.

I did not carry out double-blind controlled studies. This was not because I am unfamiliar with this technique: when I was Director of

Psychiatric Research in Saskatchewan, our group completed the first double-blind controlled experiments in psychiatry, beginning in 1953. The method was described in 1954 and the results on schizophrenic patients were reported in 1957. Two previous prospective, randomized, double-blind controlled experiments in all of medicine were completed several years before, the first in England called a double dummy experiment and the second in the USA. We compared the therapeutic effect of niacin, niacinamide, and placebo on acute schizophrenic patients. We described the technique that we had used to test a nucleotide preparation for chronic schizophrenia patients, and we were among the first to recognize the limitations of this method.

In 1970 I was called by the Director of M.D. Anderson Hospital in Texas, a well-known cancer treatment hospital. The Director asked me if I was still of the opinion I had expressed in my report to the *Canadian Medical Association Journal* where I had criticized the use of double-blind methodology. I replied that I was. He then added he and his staff of statisticians had examined my arguments over the past six months and they had concluded that I was right. The National Cancer Institute had been pressing them to do double-blind controlled experiments on their patients, but the hospital did not want to do so. He then invited me to participate in a meeting of the National Cancer Institute held in Puerto Rico where I would present my views. I was pleased to accept and attended that meeting. At a meeting in Vancouver in September 1996 I was told by a surgeon who had received his post-graduate training at this hospital that they still would not do blind clinical studies. I hope my paper had something to do with this wise decision.

It is very difficult to prepare a placebo for either ascorbic acid or sodium ascorbate when they have to be taken in large quantities. Too many capsules or tablets would be needed. I would not give my patients an equivalent amount of any of the substances commonly used for placebos. Ascorbic acid is very sour, even though it is a weak organic acid, and the ascorbate salts tend to be salty or bitter. In addition, few patients relish swallowing a large number of pills each day. It is relatively easy to prepare a placebo for anything when only small doses are needed, but not for large doses.

Patients do not like to cooperate in a double-blind experiment. Ideally in a double-blind experiment, patient and evaluating physician do not know which patient received the placebo and which received the treatment. They might not have even known that such an experiment was being conducted. Obviously, this was impossible for me. It is unethical to withhold this information from patients and perhaps even to withhold it from the clinicians. Patients would in most cases lose confidence in the clinician and in the treatment. Why should any person take a compound in large amounts daily when he or she knows that the clinician is so unsure of the efficacy that he is unwilling to place his medical reputation on the line to support the treatment? Nor will he or she relish the idea of taking large amounts of an inert substance that has no therapeutic value and may have side effects. Today, patients are much more sophisticated than they were several decades ago.

Nevertheless, I have tried to complete two double-blind experiments on my depressed patients in my private practice. They were all taking one of the current tricyclic antidepressants. I hoped to compare this drug with a similar new antidepressant. I was convinced that it would not make my patients worse, might even be more effective, and might have fewer side effects. This I explained very carefully to my patients, assuring them that they would not be made worse, might be a lot better, and would not have to pay for the experimental drug. If they were doubtful, I would not accept them into the study. I was sure that once they agreed to participate, I would have no difficulty completing the study. To my amazement I was unable to complete the study because too many patients dropped out – they did not keep their appointments. The drop-out rate from this group was much higher than it was before they started the study. My patients told me, by not coming back, that they did not trust the double-blind method and did not trust me anymore. I have not needed to be told again what they think of these experimental procedures, and have not tried to carry out such a double-blind study with cancer patients.

Moreover, it was not possible to insist that patients be seen frequently and regularly, as is called for in double-blind experiments. It would have been too costly for patients, for insurance companies, and for health insurance plans. Further, it is my experience that patients do not enjoy visiting doctors, especially when they are well.

In sum, I believe that the validity of the double-blind method has been grossly overvalued. It has only limited utility. In my opinion it does not reliably prove that effective treatments are effective and ineffective ones are ineffective. Elsewhere I had examined the reasons why it is such a limited method. The main reason is that it violates the doctor-patient relationships and therefore creates a model that is too far removed from the real clinical relationships. Not so long ago, zoologists studied the behavior of animals in a cage or even a zoo. Now they know that very limited information is obtained in this way about their natural behavior in their natural habitat. The double-blind method is to actual clinical practice what the study of monkeys in a cage is to their behavior in the forest.

Finally, double-blind experiments influence the medical-political world only when they are conducted by and reported by establishment institutions and published in establishment journals. Other double-blind experiments of equal or even greater worth unsupported by the establishment are ignored. Most clinicians know this. But research scientists also know that they will not get research grants and not be allowed to publish their results unless they are done and reported double-blind. The real reason for the popularity of the double-blinds are political, not based on scientific merit.

There is some evidence that the medical scientific world is beginning to question the dogma of the double-blind methodology, with more attention being given to controlled experiments which are not double blind. For example, Bill Moyers, in his book *Healing and The Mind*, asked Dr Dean Ornish if he had used double-blind methodology in his heart disease experiments and studies. Dr Ornish replied that the experiments he had completed were not double-blind controlled, nor were they random. He had called for volunteers from a group of patients who had just had an angiogram. Of this group half volunteered. The experimental lifestyle program included a very low fat diet, stress management, group therapy, and physical fitness exercise. Forty-seven percent of the control group improved, but, according to Dr Ornish, only if they changed their lifestyle. His experiments are now considered conclusive and have been well received.

Thus, the fact that the studies reported in this book were not double-blind controlled does not mean that the patient case histories were not studied appropriately. In most cases, each patient was studied as a series of N=1 – that is, comparisons were made of standard treatment without the orthomolecular approach against the same standard treatment combined with orthomolecular treatment. If a disease has not been controlled by treatment and will cause the death of the patient if it remains untreatable, and if something is done to the patient that changes the pattern of the illness, one can assume that what was done to the patient has altered the course of the illness. This must be the main conclusion until a better explanation is put forward – that is, one that accounts for the phenomenon more appropriately. If a series of patients are treated in the same way and there is a major shift in the course of the illness in all or a portion of the patients, then the probability that the change in course was due to other factors becomes less and less. Every control is required to test the hypothesis that treatment X did, in fact, alter the course of disease Y, so that the outcome that would have been death will be death postponed for a significant number of years.

Historical controls are helpful for they distill the natural history of a disease. If we know that every AIDS patient who is not treated will die within five years, then any treatment that increases longevity to ten or fifteen years is superior to no treatment. The main criticism of historical controls is that in time there is drift in intensity or virulence of a disease. The death rate from syphilis when it first swept through Europe was very high, but it decreased substantially after several generations.

The natural control group is the one that is used in this study. It is natural because I did not plan to have a control. Most of these patients were treatment failures, for whom there was no conventional therapy expected to be more than palliative. I had planned for everyone to be given the full benefit of orthomolecular treatment. I hoped that all the patients with cancer would want to receive this treatment and would accept this advice with the support of their physicians who had referred them to me. I played no role in providing conventional treatment directed against the cancer: surgery, irradiation, or chemotherapy. But it became clear that not every patient wanted to, or could, follow the program. It was not possible to determine in advance who would or would not follow the program. One patient was very skeptical and convinced me that she was really not very interested. Once I realized that she was not interested, I advised her not to follow the program. However, to my surprise she did follow it carefully. With several patients I was sure that they would, but they could not, or did not want to. I also had nothing to do with referrals made to my by the physicians.

The group who did not follow the program constitute a group against which to compare those who did follow the program. This group also provides an estimate of the degree of pathology present in the total group. In the majority of cases, the prognosis was poor, and this was confirmed by the death rate of the control group.

The "could not" group included patients who died before they had been on the program for two months, or who stopped following the program before they had been on it for two months. The patients who died are included in the control since they were all continuing on standard treatment of one type or another. Often it was the standard treatment that made it impossible for them to remain on my regimen. Thus, patients receiving chemotherapy were too nauseated and sick to take the nutrients in the quantities that were recommended. In my experience with megavitamin treatment, going back to 1955, I have concluded that, in most cases, it takes at least two months of treatment before the program becomes fully operative. Any period of treatment less than that would not be a fair assessment of the program. In the same way, if chemotherapy for a cancer required eight treatments over a period of several months, one could not call a treatment a failure if only one chemotherapy session were given. It would be the same as a surgeon who would remove only one quarter of the cancer from a breast and then later claim that the treatment had failed. The failure would have been the surgeon's for not following the proper surgical regimen.

As a specialist in psychiatry, I do not see primary patients, but only patients who are referred to me by other physicians. The 134 cancer patients who were referred to me during the period 1976 to 15 April 1988 were offered treatment by me for their anxiety, depression, or other psychiatric problems – the treatment that I had for decades been giving to my psychiatric patients. One quarter of the patients did not follow the regimen; they constitute the group of controls.

During the first interview I obtained the patient's history and mental state. Physical examination was done by the patient's physician, the general practitioner, the oncologist, or the surgeon. There is a psychotherapy for cancer patients. This must include a discussion of the cancer and its relationship to the immune system. Attention is given to the patient's psychiatric state and attitude, and to the use of self-help techniques such as visualization and relaxation. The nutrition that is most apt to improve their chance for recovery is outlined in some detail. The nutrients to be used are gone over carefully with respect to dose, reason for use, and possible side effects. Patients are reassured that the program will not interfere with any treatment suggested to them by their physician or oncologist. On the contrary, orthomolecular treatment decreases the toxicity of the irradiation or chemotherapy on normal tissues, increases the destructive power of the treatments on tumor tissue, and causes surgical patients to heal faster after oration, although many physicians are unaware of the large medical literature which establishes these protective and healing properties of these nutrients.

One month later the patients were seen again. Thereafter their psychiatric state and their own wishes determined whether any more interviews were needed. If they wished to see me again after six months, they would have to be re-referred by their general practitioners.

Most of the patients were residents of Vancouver Island; a few came from the city of Vancouver. All were referred for a variety of reasons. In most cases, patients requested referral after they learned that there was no use receiving any more standard treatment. Many had to consult several physicians before they found one willing to refer them. A few doctors initiated referrals. The ratio of patient-generated referrals to physician-generated referrals was very high at first, but over the past five years the ratio has been decreased significantly as more physicians are initiating the referrals. Physicians were concerned that the referral might be deemed inappropriate for patients with cancer, but can anyone visualize a patient, who knows that their life is under serious threat, not being anxious, depressed, and very concerned? In my opinion every cancer patient should be seen by a psychiatrist knowledgeable about cancer for counseling and support. In every case, continuing care was the responsibility of the referring physician and oncologist. The Cancer Clinic, when they knew their patients were taking vitamins, tried to persuade them not to. In a few cases the unhappiness was recorded in the clinical records of the clinic. Patients heard about this treatment from other patients, from their doctors, or from members of a Cancer Victors' society. There was no publicity, no press conferences, no ads, no discussion on radio or television.

– Abram Hoffer

One way in which medical progress occurs is through observations of patients made by a thoughtful physician. An example of such progress is the control of puerperal septicemia (invasion of the blood stream by bacteria in women after childbirth), which was a scourge around 150 years ago. The American poet and essayist Oliver Wendell Homes (1809-1894), author of the *The Autocrat of the Breakfast Table*, was also a physician. He was horrified by the high death rate of women in the Boston area after they had given birth to a child. He noticed that the distinguished Boston doctors, in their frock coats, went from one woman delivering a child to another without washing their hands, and he concluded that the doctors were carrying the disease from patient to patient. After publication of his book *Contagiousness of Puerperal Fever* in 1843 he was subjected to bitter abuse, which he endured with dignity. Ignacz Semmelweiss, M.D. (1818-1865), then in Vienna, stated that doctors and medical students should wash their hands in chlorinated lime water between deliveries to prevent carrying the disease from one woman to another. Within two years the death rate in his clinic had fallen from 16 percent to 1 percent. Reactionary physicians rejected his ideas for some years, and he was driven from his position in Vienna in 1849. He died in Hungary, embittered and insane, in 1865.

Another example is the medical history of the drug quinine, which is effective in preventing and treating malaria. Native Americans in Peru had discovered that chewing the bark of cinchona trees had value in controlling malarial fevers, and in 1638 this treatment was given to the wife of the Governor of Peru. The knowledge of the effectiveness of this treatment rapidly spread to Europe, and by 1820 the pure substance quinine had been isolated by chemists and was being used to control malaria.

There was no doubt about the medical value of these discoveries. Often, however, physicians or other people think that they have reason to believe in the value of a treatment that later studies show to have little or no value. Examples in the field of surgery are removal of tonsils (tonsillectomy) and of the uterus (hysterectomy), which were carried out far more often 50 to 80 years ago than now. Bypass operations for alleviation of heart disease have recently been popular, but their value for many patients is now being questioned. Many remedies or treatments of cancer have been proposed. Some of them clearly have value for some kinds of cancer, but the value of others remains in doubt.

Sometimes a treatment is used by a physician despite his knowledge that it has no value. An example is provided by a recent report of a Mayo Clinic study of 100 patients with advanced colorectal cancer. The authors state in their report that "in our opinion there is no known form of chemotherapy for colorectal cancer that had been demonstrated to provide substantive palliative benefit or extension of survival." Yet in the same report they state that "somewhat more than half the patients who have discontinued participation in this study (58 of 98) have received subsequent chemotherapy. Most of these have been treated with fluorouracil either alone or in combination with other agents." This use of chemotherapy runs counter to their earlier statement that chemotherapy has no value for these patients.

A different sort of example is the use of large doses of vitamin C in the treatment of cancer patients. Despite the evidence about its value, most physicians reject the use of vitamin C, as an adjunct to appropriate conventional therapies, for this purpose. This rejection seems to be mainly the result of ignorance of the facts.

These situations raise the following question: If a proposed treatment might have some value, but not such great value as to be obvious to everyone, how can the question of the amount of its value be answered in a convincing way?

It is for this and other purposes that the field of mathematics called biostatistics has been developed. For example, 100 patients with a certain kind of cancer at a certain stage (called a cohort of 100 patients) are entered into a study. (They might all have breast cancer in what the physicians believe to be the terminal stage, during which they receive good nursing care and drugs to control pain, when needed.) They are observed until the date of death. Their treatment, whatsoever it is, should not be changed during the time that they are in the trial. If the treatment for a patient is changed, the patient discontinues participation in the trial; that is, he or she drops out of the cohort. Mathematicians have developed a way of accounting for the fact that some patients may drop out, something they call Kaplan-Meier renormalization. At the end of the trial, when all or many of the patients have died, a study is made of their survival times, the time between entry of the patient into the trial and his or her death.

A similar trial is carried out with another cohort of 100 patients, treated in a different way. For example, the first trial might have been with terminal breast-cancer patients who received no therapeutic treatment and the second trial with similar patients who took 12 grams of vitamin C per day during the whole course of the trial.

There are several ways of comparing two trials of this sort. One way is to arrange all the patients (who have died) in the two cohorts in a single column in the order of their survival times. If all of one cohort have short survival times (low values of their rank in the column) and all of the other cohort have large survival times (high values of their rank), and if the two cohorts are truly similar, it is likely that the treatment of the second cohort is more effective than that of the first in extending survival time. Usually the two cohorts overlap in the survival-time rank. The biostatisticians have developed mathematical equations giving the reliability of the statement that, on the basis of this test, one treatment is better than the other. The equations might permit the statement to be made with 95 percent confidence, 99 percent confidence, or 99.9 percent confidence, for example.

If the two cohorts are patients in the same hospital, treated by the same physicians, there is a good likelihood of their being closely similar. Cohorts from different hospitals may be compared but with some caution.

Sometimes the patient does not know what the treatment is – capsules of an undisclosed content may be taken. The trial is then a blind trial. If also the physicians do not know what the capsules for the individual patient contain, it is called a double-blind trial. If the patients are assigned to one cohort or the other in a random way, the trials are said to be randomized.

The first randomized double-blind trials were carried out about 40 years ago. They have provided some interesting and valuable results. There are, however, also situations such that good double-blind trials cannot be carried out. A double-blind trial does not permit the treatment to be adjusted to the individual patient. For example, vitamin C has a laxative action, different for different patients. Because of this effect and for other reasons, 33 of Dr Hoffer's 134 cancer patients in our first study were unable to or refused to take any vitamin C and other nutrients; the other 101 took between 3 and 40 grams of vitamin C per day and also vitamin B-3, vitamin E, and other orthomolecular substances.

The analysis of clinical trials involving cancer patients is simplified by the existence of a general rule about their death rate that was discovered

FIGURE 1
Effect of Orthomolecular Treatment on Survival of Cancer Patients

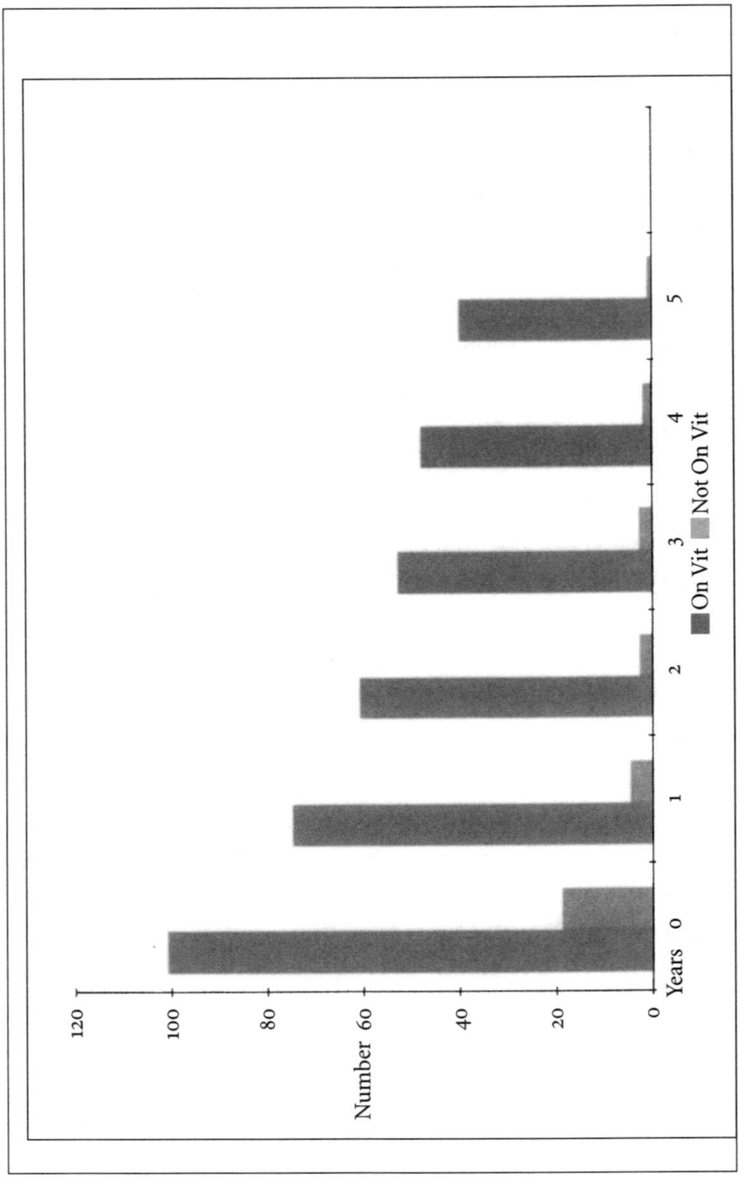

by Professor Hardin Jones, a biostatistician in the University of California, Berkeley. He was examining the survival times of reasonably homogeneous cohorts of cancer patients, and found that for many of these cohorts the chance of dying was constant; that is, during the first week a certain fraction, say 1 percent, would die, during the second week 1 percent of the survivors would die, and so on. After 69 weeks only half would remain alive, and after 138 weeks only one quarter. A survival curve can then be drawn from these facts. As Hardin Jones pointed out, this sort of survival curve is most easily recognized when the logarithm of the fraction surviving is shown as a function of time.

The analysis of the observed survival times of the 134 patients in the study made by Dr Hoffer is made complicated by the fact that 50 were still living on 1 January 1990, the termination date of the first study. A method of estimating how long these patients would probably, on the average, continue to survive was then developed on the basis of the Hardin Jones principle. It is described in an article by Abram Hoffer and Linus Pauling that was first published in the *Journal of Orthomolecular Medicine* and is reprinted in Appendix 1 of this book. The following analysis of Dr Hoffer's observations on 134 patients is based on this biostatistical method, which we believe to be reliable.

– Linus Pauling

Survival Rates

In order to obtain a comparison group for analyzing results of the orthomolecular treatment, we used the 33 patients from the original series of 134 who had not followed the program for at least two months. I had divided the group previously used as a control into two: (1) the group who did not live for two months after they first saw me – there were 14 and they lived an average 51 days; (2) the group who lived longer than two months and did not start on the vitamin program, of whom there were 19. They were alive an average of 458 days or 15 months. The first group represents a terminal group who had failed to respond to standard treatment, or who had suffered a relapse after an initial response to previous treatment, and who may have been compromised by the treatment they had already received. It would have been desirable for patients who had decided for personal reasons never to accept any xenobiotic therapy to become a control group, but this was simply not possible in this study, nor would I recommend this to my patients for ethical reasons. As well, it is quite likely that some of the 101 patients in the treated group would also have died within that two month interval had they not been started on orthomolecular therapy, but this cannot be determined for these patients. Perhaps an equal number lived longer than two months as did those who did not make it for the two months after they first saw me. Taking all these factors into account, I think it is fair and reasonable to use the second control group as another valid comparison group, a concurrent group. This should also satisfy critics who maintain that every patient entered into the study must be retained in it, even if they did not follow the treatment protocol.

Using this comparison group, there were 101 patients who were able to follow the program, although some of them did not live very long after I first saw them. None were excluded from this group. The results of the treatment on the 101 can be compared with the results of the xenobiotic treatment on the 19. I now have over 770 patients in my series. I found that the difference between the vitamin treated patients and those who were not on the program was sustained. Survival of the two groups, the treated group of 101 and the pseudo-control group of 19 treated only with xenobiotic therapy, are shown in Figure 1.

The difference in outcome between these two groups remained large. In the first year, 75 percent of the group not on the orthomolecular program died, and at the end of five years 5 percent were alive. From the orthomolecular group, 25 percent died by the end of the first year, and at the end of the fifth year, 39 percent were alive. By January 1, 1992, 41 patients were still alive. The average duration of life from the time I first saw them until this date was 49 months, compared to 15 months for the group treated with xenobiotic therapy only.

As Dr Pauling has observed, "based on the results so far, I predict that they will live 5 to 7 years. So many are still alive that it's hard to predict how long they'll live." The mean survival time estimate for both groups is about 80 months. The survival of the xenobiotic group resembled much more closely our original group of 33. Therefore, even with this control group which contains all the patients who followed the program for as little as a few days, the outcome of treatment was still supportive of our conclusion

FIGURE 2

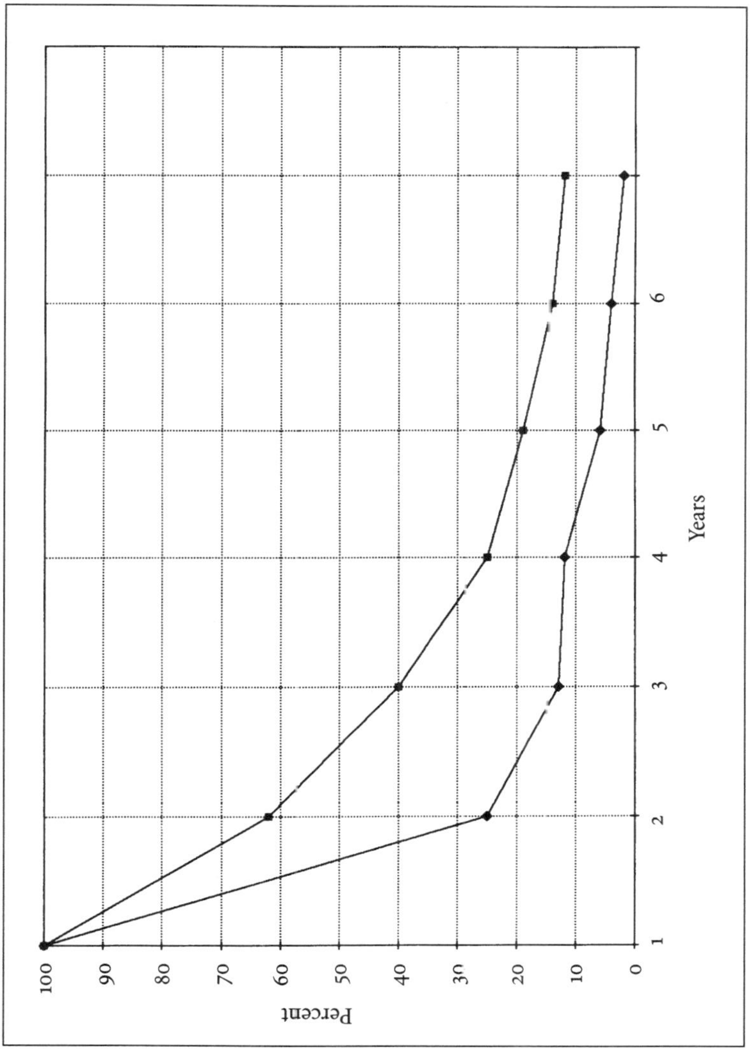

Comparison of Adjunctive (Orthomolecular and Standard) Against Standard Treatment Adjunctive Upper (N=457), Standard Lower (N=52)

that orthomolecular treatment combined with xenobiotic treatment is much superior to xenobiotic therapy alone. As a clinician working with patients for 42 years, I still think the original control group is the sounder one to use scientifically.

Twenty patients out of 59 (34 percent) survived 8 years. They were first seen between 1978 and 1984. From the remaining 75, seen between 1985 and 1988, 22 (29 percent) survived four years. This suggests that over the next four years this group will also yield a 25 percent, 8-year survival. The first group included the following types of cancers: pancreas (1), lung (2), sarcoma (2), lymphoma (3), throat (2), uterus (2), ovary (1), breast (5), cervix (1), and colon (1).

Another way to compare the effect of orthomolecular against the standard therapy is to eliminate every patient I have seen who did not survive two months after I first saw them. Following this method, I have examined the survival by years of 562 patients all seen from 1978 to February 24, 1994. From this group, there were 457 on orthomolecular treatment and 52 who were not. The latter is the control group and represents the results of standard treatment they had been getting from the time they first were diagnosed. This data is to be used only to compare these two treatments; it cannot be used to predict the outcome of treatment since many of the patients were seen too recently. But it does show that arbitrarily removing patients from the treated group who have not been on the program at least two years will not distort the data showing what the final outcome will be, as shown in Figure 2.

Cancer Types

A comparison of the survival rates among patients involved in this study according to the type of cancer shows that the same proportion of breast cancer, prostate cancer, and colon cancer were alive after 10 years. Lung cancer patients, the only other group with a significant number, had a poor prognosis with a very small 5 to 10 year survival. The ovarian cancer group had the worst response record. The best responders were the lymphomas and the uterine cancers, but both these groups were small. The mean 5 to 10 year survivals are shown in Table 6.

Staging and Survival

Staging for the tumors in these patients was the responsibility of the treating physicians using standard treatments. The clinical files and reports I was able to obtain in most cases did not contain the stages of the illness. Most of the patients were late in their illness and undoubtedly would have been staged by the time I first saw them as Stage 4. But as I was not the first to see and diagnose them, they might have been classified differently at the time of first diagnosis, which most often occurred some time before I saw them and before treatment was started. It was not possible for me to estimate from the files what would have been the staging at the time of first diagnosis when staging is most appropriate. It is possible to obtain an estimate of the severity of the disease by comparing the outcome of the group not on the orthomolecular regimen with the outcome for these types of tumors available in the literature. The two main groups were not randomly selected for this study, but there was a lot of randomness in the selection which was done by the patients themselves, or by the nature of the treatment they received, or by the fact a few could not live long enough to benefit from treatment.

In the *Manual for Staging of Cancer*, 10-year survival rates are given for colorectal cancer, for lung cancer, and for breast cancer. In my series, colorectal and breast cancer have nearly the same 5 to 10-year survival rate as the average for the whole group. With colorectal cancers, the survival data is closest to the Stage 4 survival curve in the *Manual* (Figure 12-1, 76). In the *Manual*, about 38 percent survive one year compared to 17 percent in my series; about 18 percent survive two years but there were none in my series. However, the outcome for the treated group was much better with nearly 40 percent living ten years. This is comparable with Stage 3 where 40 percent lived for ten years. In other words, the addition of the vitamin regimen improved the outcome from worse than one would expect with Stage 4 patients when first diagnosed to the outcome expected of Stage 3 patients. The non-treated group represents an estimate of the mean overall staging of the entire series.

Similar results are seen for the breast cancer patients. The smaller group not receiving the orthomolecular regimen had a survival curve below the Stage 4 curve shown in the *Manual* (Fig 25-1, 151), while the treated group survival curve was very close to the one shown for Stage 3 patients. And for the entire group the comparison non-treated group survival curve was worse than that shown for Stage 4 breast and colorectal cancer. The treated group had a survival pattern very similar to the one found for Stage 3 breast cancer. It is interesting that in the survival curves published the survival decreases year by year without reaching a plateau. With our orthomolecular series, a plateau is reached at about 4 to 5 years and remains relatively stable for the next 5 years. These comparisons are consistent with the conclusion that the use of a nutritional supplement approach improves the outcome of cancer treatment, not just for the first 5 years of follow up but for another 5 years.

– Abram Hoffer

Biostatistical Analysis of the Survival Rates

Before making a more detailed analysis of the results of this study of the effect of orthomolecular treatment on cancer for the first series of 134 patients involved in this study, we may ask a simple question: What fraction of the patients who followed the orthomolecular regimen were still alive at the termination of the first study, 31 December 1989, and what fraction of those who did not follow the regimen were still alive at that time?

Admission into the first study ended on 15 April 1988, so that the length of survival of the survivors was at least 18 months. There was no difference in the times of entry into the study: by 1 January 1986, 52 percent of those who followed the regimen and 48 percent of the others had entered the study. The number of survivors at the closing of the study was 48 out of 101 (48 percent) for those who followed the regimen and only 2 out of 33 (6 percent) for the others. This is an astonishing result. Considering the fact that the regimen does not involve any drugs or physical treatment (such as high-energy radiation) and cannot be considered in itself to be dangerous or harmful, it is hard to see why every cancer patient should not at once be put on the regimen.

A more thorough analysis gives even more striking results. The careful study reported in Appendix I (Hardin Jones Biostatistical Analysis of Mortality Data for Cohorts of Cancer Patients...) leads to the conclusion that the 31 controls constituting Tables 1 and 2 (excluding two longer-lived patients, each of whom had a kind of cancer not represented by any other patient) had a mean survival time of 5.7 months, as expected for patients with advanced cancer. The 101 patients who followed the regimen seem to be divided into a group of 20 poor responders, with mean survival time 10 months, only about twice that of the controls, and a much larger group of 81 excellent responders, with a mean survival time of 92 months, 16 times that of the controls. Further information about survival of patients with different kinds of cancer who followed the orthomolecular regimen can also be obtained from the data in the tables in Appendix 1. For this comparison, we make the assumption that for each small group of patients with a particular kind of cancer listed in Table 4 in the Appendix, the excellent responders have t = 122 months, with t = 72 months for the excellent responders listed in Table 5. The number of patients who lived only 20 months or less can be used to determine the fraction of patients constituting the excellent responders for each kind of cancer. These fractions range from 73 percent to 100 percent, possibly reliable to ± 5percent. An effort was made also to evaluate the mean expected survival time for the excellent responders with different kinds of cancer but it failed because the number of patients is too small.

Cancer of the Breast

Of the 26 breast-cancer patients who followed the orthomolecular regimen, with 17 (63 percent) alive at the end of the study, 92 percent (25) constitute the excellent responders, with a mean expected survival time of 122 months, 34 times the mean observed survival time of the five controls, 3.6 months. There is no evidence that the controls differ in any significant way from the patients who followed the regimen, except that they did not receive the vitamins and other nutrients. The conclusion that the 26 patients benefitted greatly from the regimen cannot be rejected. By the end of June 1996, 11 were still alive, and 14 had lived at least 7 years.

Evidence about the state of the disease on entry of the patients into the study is provided by the number of lymph nodes that had been invaded by metastatic malignant cells and by other information. The 32 women with breast cancer who entered this study constituted a very sick group, as must be inferred from the following clinical observations. Only two (6 percent) had not had surgery before being registered for the orthomolecular regimen of treatment. Symptoms and signs had been present for an average of

14 months before entry into the study (range 1 to 48 months). In most of the patients the conventional treatment had failed, and the orthomolecular regimen was started after surgery, irradiation, and chemotherapy. For only two patients was surgery carried out at about the time that the orthomolecular regimen was begun. Only two breast-cancer patients were classified as having reached Stage 1 or Stage 2 at entry into the study, with 24 in Stage 3 and Stage 4, and no information for 6. (Stage 1, tumor diameter less than 2 cm; Stage 2, diameter 2 to 5 cm; Stage 3, diameter greater that 5 cm, tumor usually attached to chest wall or skin, few metastases; Stage 4, same as Stage 3, plus more metastases.)

The reported numbers of lymph nodes are 0 to 6 for treated patients and 1 control, 1 to 3 for 6 treated patients and 1 control, and 4 to 12 for 7 treated patients and 2 controls. For the patients who followed the orthomolecular regimen, the fraction alive at the termination of the study decreases from 100 percent to 43 percent as the number of affected nodes increase, and the mean expected survival time also decreases somewhat. These observations suggest that the orthomolecular regimen is somewhat more effective in the earlier course of the advanced disease than the later course, and emphasizes the importance of taking the megavitamins as early as possible.

Cancer of the Uterus

Of the 8 patients with cancer of the uterus (including the uterine cervix) who followed the regimen, with 4 alive at the end of the study, 73 percent constitute the group of excellent responders, with mean expected survival time, 122 months, 31 times the mean survival time of the single control, 4 months. The four patients who were alive at the end of this study are still alive on June 31, 1996, over 10 years each (120 months).

Cancer of the Ovary

Of 9 patients with ovarian cancer, 5 accepted the regimen and 4 did not. We find that 61 percent of those who followed the regimen (1 alive at the end of the study) are excellent responders, with mean expected survival time, 122 months, 22 times that of the 4 controls, 5.5 months. From the orthomolecular group, 2 lived 2 years and one is alive after 10 years.

Cancer of the Lung

Of the 14 patients with lung cancer, 11 followed the orthomolecular regimen, and 8 were still living at the end of the study. About 65 percent of the patients constitute the excellent responders, with mean expected survival time of 72 months, 16 times the mean survival time, 3.3 months, of the 3 patients who did not follow the regimen. Of the 8 one-year survivors, 5 lived 2 years, 3 lived 3 years, 2 lived 10 years, and one was still alive after 12 years. The actual survival for this group is just over 50 months.

Cancer of the Colon, Bowel, Abdomen, and Intestine

Of the 10 patients with cancer of the colon, bowel, abdomen, or intestine (4 alive at the end of the study) who followed the regimen, the group of excellent responders constitutes 73 percent with mean expected survival time of 72 months, 14 times the mean survival time, 5.3 months of the 5 controls. In June 1996 the same 4 are still alive. The mean survival time is 80 months.

Cancer of the Pancreas

There are 4 patients with cancer of the pancreas who followed the regimen (2 alive at the end of the study) and only 1 who did not. The analysis led to the conclusion that about 74 percent (3 of the 4) can be assigned to the excellent responder group, with mean expected survival time taken to be 72 months, 30 times that of the single control, 2.4 months. This ratio is, of course, unreliable. If the single control had survived the average time for controls, 5.7 months, the value of the ratio would have been only 13.

Even this ratio is surprisingly high for patients with cancer of the pancreas. This kind of cancer is considered by oncologists to be untreatable by any conventional therapy, with survival time after diagnosis never as long as five years. Yet one of the patients, a woman who followed the orthomolecular regimen, taking between 14 and 40 grams of ascorbic acid per day as well as other nutrients, had survived for 137 months (over 11 years) by the end of the study and remained in good health in June 1996.

There is no doubt that the effect of the orthomolecular regimen on patients with cancer of the pancreas is highly beneficial. Dr Mao et al reported cancer survival rates for Alberta, Canada, for the years 1974 to

1978. Only 3 percent of female patients with cancer of the pancreas lived three years, and no one lived five years. R. Falk and associates compared the effect of radiofrequency hyperthermia and chemotherapy with and without immune stimulation in a group of 77 patients with adenocarcinoma of the pancreas. In the first group, no patient survived longer than 21 months, and in the immune-stimulated group, 14 percent survived 42 months, but none more than 45 months.

Other Kinds of Cancer

For the 14 other kinds of cancer, the numbers of patients are small. At the present time it may not be unreasonable to expect for them about the same values as for those discussed above, about an 80 percent chance for those following the orthomolecular regimen of being in the excellent-responder group, with expected mean survival times about 72 months.

In summary, it is our opinion that the survival times of cancer patients depend greatly on the daily intake of vitamin C and other vitamins, and to some extent minerals, such a selenium. The difference in survival times between mega amounts and the usual intake for patients with advanced cancer has now been shown to be very great by the work of Ewan Cameron and his associates, F. Morishige, and the present study. So far as mega amounts of vitamin C are concerned, it is our opinion that larger amounts, 12 grams per day or more, up to the bowel tolerance limit, are more effective than somewhat smaller amounts, 3 g/day to 6 g/d. The number of patients in the present study is, however, too small to provide evidence on this point.

– Linus Pauling

Follow-Up Studies

In my 1994 report on our study, I examined further the first cohort of 134 patients as of December 1993. Thirty-four were still alive from the treated group, all having survived at least five years. None survived from the control group. Seventeen survived more than 10 years. As of July 1994 another 17 patients are alive. Four will reach 10 years in 4 years, 7 in 3 years, 4 in 2 years and 2 in 2 years. I expect that there will be 34 who will have reached a 10-year survival. Half the 6 deaths in 1992 died of other physical disease, not directly from their cancer. One died in 1993.

TABLE 7

Treatments Given to 10-Year Survivors

#	Born	Sex	Organ	Surg	Rad	Chemo	Start
1	1920	F	Lung	No	Yes	No	04/84
11	1959	M	Lymphoma	Yes	Yes	Yes	03/84
18	1917	M	Vocal Cords	Yes	Yes	No	06/80
19	1943	F	Uterus	Yes	Yes	No	02/83
22	1965	F	Ewing Sarc	No	Yes	Yes	08/81
23	1941	F	Ovary	Yes	Yes	Yes	05/82
27	1937	F	Breast	Yes	Yes	No	12/83
35	1926	F	Breast	Yes	Yes	Yes	11/82
37	1927	F	Lung	No	Yes	Yes	03/81
60	1946	F	Cervix	No	No	No	03/83
62	1935	F	Breast	Yes	No	No	06/83
66	1970	F	Lymphoma	Yes	No	Yes	02/84
74	1947	M	Lymphoma	Yes	Yes	Yes	06/83
84	1919	F	Pancreas	Yes	No	No	07/78
86	1941	M	Throat	Yes	Yes	No	03/81
87	1952	M	Colon	Yes	No	No	04/82
91	1911	F	Uter&thyr	Yes	Yes	Yes	05/80

At the Tulsa conference in 1992, I examined the first cohort of 134 further after describing what was the orthomolecular regimen that I used. In the first year after treatment, 75 percent of the control group of 33 died compared to 25 percent from the treated group of 101. On 1 January 1992, 41 patients were still alive from the treated group and one from the control. The average survival was 49 months for the treated group compared to 15 months for the control. The survival data suggested that the original Hoffer and Pauling estimates of survival were not far off the mark.

At another conference in San Diego in March 1994, I reported on what happened to the first 134 patient cohort as of 31 December 1993; 34 were still alive from the treated group and none from the controls.

Patients Alive After Ten Years

Seventeen patients from the treated cohort of 101 lived at least ten years after treatment was started. In the following table I have shown some of the treatment variables. Only one was treated by orthomolecular treatment alone. The remainder had the usual standard treatments as determined by their own physicians and the cancer clinic they had attended. The proportion of all the patients receiving these therapies is the same as it is for this smaller group of survivors.

With any individual patient predictions about the future are bound to be very uncertain even for diseases with a very poor track record. But for some diseases death is so certain that every survival beyond what is expected must be considered important. Thus it is relevant to get an estimate of the severity of the disease. For each of the 10-year survivors I will indicate the evidence that they were examples of cancer with a poor prognosis. When the number of such cases begins to add up, the data becomes more and more relevant. I have used the following lines of evidence to indicate prognosis. (1) Conclusions by oncologists and surgeons that the prognosis is poor. They have made these predictions on the basis of their expertise in treating similar cancers using orthodox methods. This includes the surgeon's opinion that the lesion was inoperable. Patients 1,11,37,66,74, and 84. (2) Recurrences of the same lesion after the original had been treated. (3) The inherent nature of the cancer – e.g., Ewings sarcoma and cancer of the pancreas. (4) Metastases and spread of the tumor beyond its original site. The pertinent evidence from these brief cases is listed below. Out of 17 long term survivors, 13 had poor prognosis. Most of them were Stage 3 and Stage 4.

Patient # 1. Lung. The Cancer Clinic found a squamous cell cancer occluding the right upper lobe of the bronchus which had collapsed the lobe and had extended laterally to the right main bronchus. She was given irradiation in 20 sessions over 4 weeks. Two years later she was free of cancer but had developed intermittent claudication. She increased the niacin to 1.5 grams daily and has remained well since. In 1988 there was no lymphadenopathy and her chest was clear. On 24 December 1993 she suffered a stroke. She died 25 January 1994 from her stroke, not from the cancer.

Patient # 11. Lymphoma. His oncologist recorded, "He presents with an incurable condition which undoubtedly in the near future will take him away." Because of his psychiatric disease, it was much more difficult for him to follow his program carefully.

Patient # 18. Vocal Cords. He needed repeated surgery to remove the tumor which kept recurring. Only after radiotherapy and starting the vitamin program did the recurrences stop.

Patient # 19. Uterus. Nine years after hysterectomy she had a carcinoma in situ in the labia. This indicated that the pressure for recurrence was still present.

Patient # 22. Ewings Sarcoma. A huge mass was present which eventually required filling in the bone.

Patient # 23. Ovary. In 1981 Papillary adenocarcinoma of the oviduct with invasion into the ovary. On 10 April 1985 she had secondaries in her bones and one tumor in her cerebellum.

Patient # 27. Breast. I have no information whether she was Stage I or II.

Patient # 35. Breast. By then some of the glands were involved and the cancer was adherent to her ribs. In 1976 another lump appeared in her right breast and was removed by lumpectomy. After that she continued to suffer small recurrent tumors which cleared.

Patient # 37. Lung. A visible tumor involving the lateral wall of the right lower lobe bronchus and extending into the right upper lobe bronchus and occluding the orifice of the superior segment of the right lower. She also had an ill defined area in the left tempero parietal region. She was considered inoperable.

Patient # 60. Cervix. After an abnormal pap smear she had three biopsies and was diagnosed as carcinoma in situ of the cervix. Her surgeon recommended hysterectomy, which she rejected.

Patient # 62. Breast. In March 1982 she had a modified radical right mastectomy, followed two weeks later by a left mastectomy because of suspicious cellular changes. A few lymph nodes were positive. She rejected any further treatment and started the vitamin regimen instead. On February 1994 she was well.

Patient # 66. Hodgkins. He developed Hodgkins lymphoma with the tumors in his abdomen. He was given a 10 percent chance of survival.

Patient # 74. Lymphoma. Diagnosed with "a small cell diffuse lymphocytic lymphoma described as controllable, not curable... clearly has a progressive disease not being controlled by chlorambucil and prednisone. However, I can definitely state that this man has persistent incurable malignant disease."

Patient # 84. Pancreas. A 6 cm in diameter hard mass was found in the head of the pancreas which totally obstructed her common bile duct. The diagnosis was so certain it was decided not to do a biopsy in order not to increase the chance of metastases. A cholecysto-jejunostomy was performed. After the operation she was informed her prognosis was very poor and that she should get her affairs in order.

Patient # 86. Throat. No evidence with respect to prognosis.

Patient # 87. Colon. The transverse section was resected. The tumor had perforated the bowel and was infected. Some of his spleen was removed. There had been no spread.

Patient # 91. Thyroid. Partial thyroidectomy, removing one half of her gland which contained an adenoma. After that she had daily deep x-ray irradiation. In 1971 she had a ileostomy for severe colitis present the previous 7 years and in 1974 a hysterectomy.

From the 17 patients in the 10-year survivor group, 13 had poor prognoses. From the group who died during the second year, all of them had a poor prognosis. One cancer of the pancreas is still alive 15 years later, but there are two others who have beaten the odds from this very malignant cancer. On 21 April 1994, one had survived for 17 months, the other for 7 years. Five patients with pancreatic cancer died within the first year. A ratio of 3 survivors out of 8 is fairly impressive. There were 26 patients with breast cancer. The number alive at years 1, 2, 3, 5, and 6 is 24, 20, 20, 15, and 15. I have examined the survival numbers from a different cohort of 59 cases of breast cancer first seen in 1988 to 1991 inclusive. Alive at 1 and 2 years were 48 and 41. These are very similar to the equivalent survivals in the original cohort of 101.

The survival trends which appeared in the first Hoffer and Pauling paper and reappeared in our second and in my third presentation were reconfirmed in this report. From 101 on the program, a core of 34 patients remain who have survived more than 5 years and from which 17 have survived more than ten years. Over half of the seven 1992 deaths died of physical factors not directly related to their cancer.

In another earlier report, I examined further the first cohort of 134 patients as of December 1993. Thirty-four were still alive from the treated

TABLE 8
The Survival By Years of All Patients on The Vitamin Regimen and on Standard Treatment Only Seen Between 1978 and the end of 1993

On Orthomolecular Plus Standard Treatment					Standard Only		
Year Seen	Years could have lived	Number at risk	Alive at end of year	Percent alive	N	Alive	%
1994	1	518	375	72	118	17	14
1993	2	440	242	55	102	8	8
1992	3	369	178	48	93	8	9
1991	4	301	132	44	82	6	7
1990	5	244	98	40	65	4	6
1989	6	185	76	41	56	2	4
1988	7	142	53	37	42	0	0
1987	8	108	41	38			
1986	9	80	31	39			
1985	10	56	22	39			

group, all having survived at least 5 years. None survived from the control group. Seventeen survived more than 10 years. Over half the 7 deaths in 1992 died of other physical disease, not directly from their cancer. One died in 1993. By the end of 1994, out of the control group of 33, 1 lived 3 years, 1 lived 4 years, and 1 lived 6 years.

The Entire Series

(N=636 Patients Seen Between 1978 and 31 December 1993)
In our first two reports on our studies, Dr Linus Pauling examined the probability of survival by using the Hardin Jones Biostatistical Method (see Appendix 1). In subsequent reports, I used the actual survival by years. With a much larger series, now 542 patients, the actual survival data becomes more meaningful. The two basic methods of examining outcome yield similar conclusions – i.e., that the patient groups on the orthomolecular regimen had a better survival outcome than did the group of patients receiving all the standard treatments but not the orthomolecular treatment.

I have examined the survival rate by years, by comparing the total number of patients at risk who could have lived one or two or more years against the number who actually did live these years. Thus 518 patients given the combined treatment and 118 who received only xenobiotic treatment were seen by the end of 1993. They could have lived the whole year. Only 375 from the first group did live one year, and 17 from the second group. By 1989 185 patients from the total treatment group were seen who could have lived five years but only 76 did. This is shown in Table 8 and displayed graphically in Figure 3.

Patients on the combined program who live more than 4 years have an excellent chance of living 10 years. The usually accepted 5-year survival rate is confirmed by this data. The control group did not do nearly as well and only 5 percent achieved a 5-year survival.

Treatments included surgery, radiation, chemotherapy, ascorbic acid, vitamin B-3, beta carotene, zinc and selenium, and various combinations. Because these groups were not randomized, it is not possible to compare accurately the various combinations against the control group. I have examined the 5-year survival data for some of the combinations, using the overall 40 percent 5-year survival as the standard. All the combinations yielded about the same 5-year survival. The major difference was in the total program compared to the standard treatment only group.

FIGURE 3
Percent Survival of All Patients

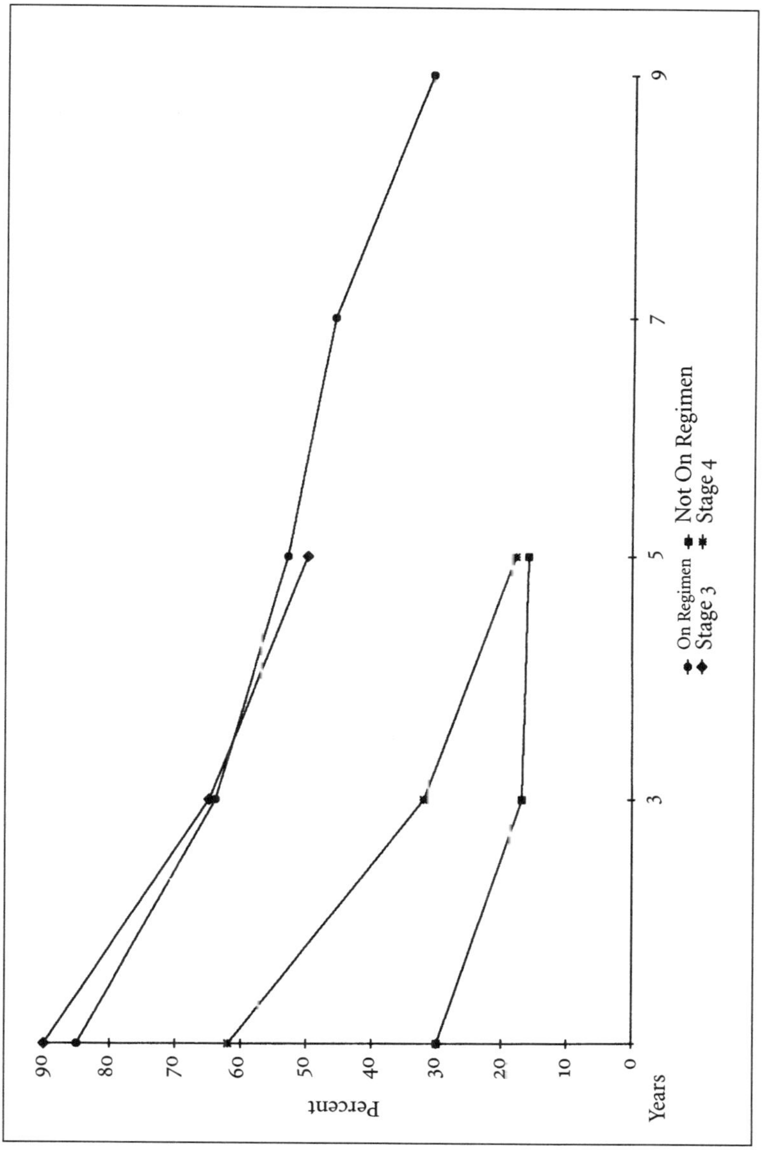

Different Xenobiotic Treatment

The one and five year survival was not affected by the various combinations of surgery, chemotherapy, and radiation that were used. Because this was not a randomized prospective study, the groups were different. The clinical decision to use the treatments was based on the nature of the lesion, its severity, whether it had spread, and age. The more complex therapies were given to patients with the worst prognosis, with the exception that if the lesion was inoperable or untreatable, few if any of these therapies were offered. Thus a patient receiving all three treatments was undoubtedly much sicker compared to one receiving only one treatment, in most cases. The fact that all the treatment combinations yielded the same follow up data suggests that the clinicians were pretty skillful in selecting the most appropriate treatment so that even the worst cases gave the same results compared to the ones where simpler therapy was followed. I did not exclude any patient and advised them all to follow the program, but, of course, many did not or could not.

The follow up data on patients who received the orthomolecular program plus surgery alone, or radiation alone, or chemotherapy alone is shown in Table 9.

The Nutrients

There was no difference between those taking or not taking beta carotene, zinc, selenium, and vitamin B-3. This suggests that with the multiple use of antioxidant nutrients dropping one does not materially decrease the

TABLE 9

Follow up Results of Surgery, Radiation, and Chemotherapy Alone Combined with Orthomolecular Therapy

Treatment	One year			Five years		
	Number could have lived	Alive	%	Number could have lived	Alive	%
Surgery only	90	68	76	32	18	56
Radiation only	44	26	59	19	7	53
Chemotherapy only	19	15	79	6	3	50

TABLE 10
The Survival By Years of All Patients on The Vitamin Regimen between 1978 and the end of 1993 by Age

		Born in 1930 or earlier			Born in 1931 or later		
Year Seen	Years could have lived	Number at risk	Alive at end of year	Percent alive	N	Alive	%
1993	1	203	134	66	235	184	78
1992	2	176	89	51	192	124	75
1991	3	149	62	42	150	83	55
1990	4	127	45	35	115	57	50
1989	5	97	37	38	86	39	45
1988	6	78	27	35	62	30	48
1987	7	60	19	32	47	23	49
1986	8	43	14	33	36	19	53
1985	9	27	7	26	28	16	58
1978 to 1984	10	24	5	21	21	14	67

response. But I have no evidence to suggest what dropping two or three would do. Of the nutrients, vitamins C plays the major one, while the addition of other antioxidants improves the results. The series is too small to examine for the absence of two or three of these antioxidants while retaining ascorbic acid. It will be necessary to use randomized prospective controls to determine the relative value of the various antioxidants.

Age

Age of the patient determines the response to this treatment approach. The effect of age is shown in Table 10 and displayed graphically in Figure 4.

The older age group did not do as well. Either they could not respond as well to treatment or they had a larger proportion dying from other causes only indirectly related to the cancer. But the younger group had an advantage even in the shorter term follow-up, suggesting that the older group were more vulnerable to their disease and more vulnerable to the toxic treatment they were given. This, I think was the main factor. About

FIGURE 4
Survival By Age

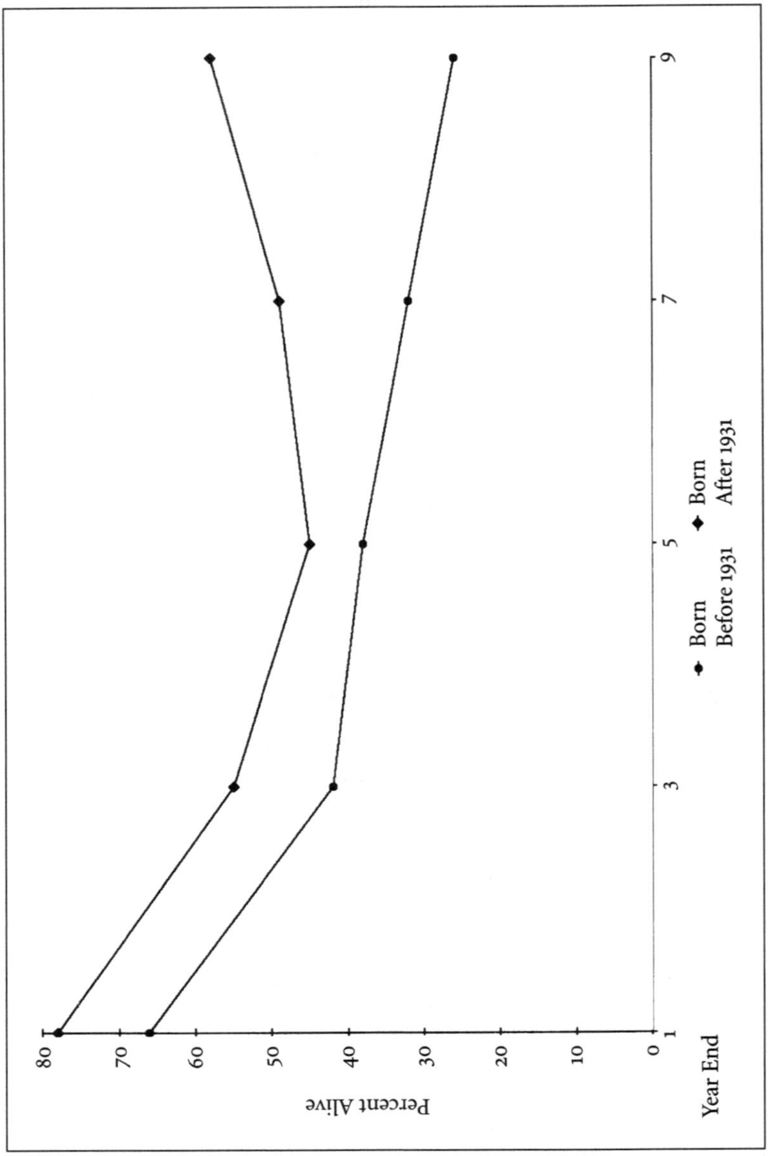

TABLE 11

All Cancer Patients on the Regimen to End of 1994

Seen by year end	Number Seen	1st	2nd	3rd	4th	5th	Percent
		Years following first visit — Alive: Number Alive					
1990	244					98	48
1991	301				132		44
1992	369			176			48
1993	480		241				58
1994	518	373					72

All Cancer Patients Not on the Regimen to End of 1994

Seen by year end	Number Seen	1st	2nd	3rd	4th	5th	Percent
		Years following first visit — Alive: Number Alive					
1990	68					4	6
1991	82				6		7
1992	93			8			9
1993	102		8				8
1994	118	17					14

35 percent of the patients in the older age group lived in the follow up period 4 to 10 years. For the younger group about 50 percent survived.

Survival of all cancer patients seen to the end of 1994 is shown in Table 11.

This conclusion applies only to patients who have received a combination of all the standard modalities of treatment with orthomolecular treatment. Better results were found with patients who were placed on the combination soon after they were diagnosed and standard treatment was started. Arbitrarily, I have concluded that there must be a minimum two-month period on the nutritional program before it can begin to demonstrate its power to prolong life. More study will be required to determine what is the minimum period.

Quality of Life

It is difficult to measure quality of life quantitatively, but it is relatively easy to find out whether the patients and their families were more comfortable, suffered less pain, and remained more functional. A large proportion of my patients in fact told me they were more comfortable, more functional, and suffered less pain. Frequently, they were able to decrease the amount of narcotic. Even when they lived for only a short time after they saw me, they felt they had benefited, and often after death, their families would let me know how grateful they were that they had suffered so much less. I have not had a single complaint from my patients that they suffered more pain and discomfort. This contrasts strongly with xenobiotic therapy which is characterized by severe discomfort of many kinds – nausea, fatigue of long duration, loss of hair, etc.

Orthomolecular therapy tends to decrease the discomfort caused by xenobiotic therapy. This is also difficult to quantify, but I believe my patients were telling me what really happened when they reported that they were able to tolerate radiation and chemotherapy better. Their surgeons often were surprised by their rapid recovery from surgery. They were discharged very quickly from hospital.

Oncologists are beginning to emphasize the importance of considering duration and quality of life in measuring response to treatment. Tumor shrinkage alone is no longer considered an adequate measure. Dr Ian Tannock, Chief of Medicine at Princess Margaret Hospital in Toronto and an oncologist, said at a recent meeting at the International Congress on Care of the Terminally Ill, "It's only recently, over the last decade or so, that people have started to realize and appreciate the importance of quality of life end points in determining what we do.... It is my thesis and strong opinion that the appropriate end points (in clinical trials) are those of patient benefit, that patients live longer and do things better."

After working with over 630 patients with cancer since 1978, I have no doubt that the megavitamin program has improved the quality of their life. It has given them more energy, has improved depression and anxiety, has created a sense of well being, has eased pain, and often has eliminated the pain entirely. A recent remarkable response will illustrate the effect of this program.

Born in 1922, this patient was first seen on 6 January 1994. She had a mastectomy in March 1990, right side. In March 1992 she developed low back pain which did not respond to chiropractic treatment or physiotherapy. In August 1992 she discovered a node in her neck. A bone scan showed two areas in the spine. She was given Tamoxifen, but after five days the pain became intolerable and she went off it against the wishes of her oncologist. After that, she started taking herbs and massage and was well in three months. In September 1993 the pain recurred. Now she had metastases in her sternum and lower back. Pain in her chest was severe. She started on Tamoxifen again, and the pain became much worse. After two weeks, she started on ascorbic acid 15 grams daily and on shark cartilage, but could only tolerate 8 capsules of the cartilage. After starting the vitamin C, she slowly began to improve. She was able to leave her bed, but she still needed morphine every 12 hours. I advised her to follow the megavitamin program which included 15 g of ascorbic acid plus Coenzyme Q_{10}, 300 mg. On 1 February 1994 she was free of pain and had discontinued the morphine. This she appreciated since the severe nausea generated by the morphine was gone. By 23 February 1994 the lumps had decreased to half their original size and she was able to move freely without pain. Both she and her husband were delighted.

Quality of life involves physical and emotional health. Physically, a large number of symptoms will seriously interfere with the enjoyment of life. These include pain, restriction of movement, inability to function – for example, to swallow – nausea and vomiting, loss of weight and appetite, ability to meet energy requirements. I consider a person has a good quality of life when these factors are not present or are present to such a limited degree that they do not interfere with one's lifestyle.

Emotional health is equally if not more important. The main changes in cancer patients when given the diagnosis are shock, depression, anxiety, and the effect this mood has upon thinking and behavior. It is generated by the diagnosis, by the way it is given to them, and by the knowledge that cancer is a major killing disease. One of the main problems is the fear shared by too many oncologists, surgeons, and radiotherapists of the peculiar combination of words "false hope." This is a basic contradiction of terms. There are various degrees of hope ranging from none to excessive. The term derives from the fear of the physicians that they will give a prognosis which is too optimistic and cannot be confirmed by follow up. They have gone to the other extreme and have been prone to give the patients zero hope. Dr William Osler, the famous Canadian-American physician, wrote about the importance of hope and to illustrate it he told the following story about himself. He was asked to examine a man who had already been examined by two physicians who had advised the family that he would die that day. The family wanted another opinion. After his examination, Dr Osler told the family that in his opinion he would not die that day. But he did die. The next morning the family approached Dr Osler and thanked him profusely. He was, they said, the only physician who had given them some hope. If there is anything at all to the placebo response, to the value of hope in the treatment of disease, then physicians must not remove this important variable. Even when it looks very grim indeed, the patient and family must be allowed some of the comforts of hope, though it must be realistic. It is essential not to exaggerate the hope. The patient should be advised that no matter how grim the situation is, there is some hope and that the physician will help in any way possible. The best way to enhance hope is to be able honestly to report about other patients equally ill who have had their lives prolonged and the quality of life improved.

As M.L. Slevin has suggested, "It is almost always negative to tell people that they have a fixed life expectancy. The averages apply to populations and not to individuals and to give people a fixed life expectancy removes hope and provokes depression and despondency. It is more appropriate and helpful to indicate that while life might be very short if things go badly, the length of life could still be long and cannot be estimated if things go well." A.M. Levine has described the effect of hope on two cancer patients. A 55-year-old woman was found to have an inoperable squamous cell carcinoma invading the mediastinal nodes. It was biopsied. The next morning the resident told her, "Well, it's cancer, and we couldn't really resect it, so we just opened and closed." She asked, "Opened and closed?" She repeated this several times. She died that night. At autopsy there was no specific cause of death. The resident had removed all hope. The second patient had an aggressive T-cell immunoblastic sarcoma. He refused chemotherapy after being informed it likely would not help much. Dr Levine, however, told him that there was a chance, albeit a slim one. He went into remission and was well for one year. Unfortunately, the cancer clinics too often leave their patients bereft of hope. Slevin also discussed the importance of providing emotional support. Patients most often wanted support from their physician and more senior doctors, not as much from nurses, psychologists, and social workers delegated to provide it. They got this support from receiving accurate and authoritative information, as they saw it.

Recently, I saw on follow up a man with lymphoma who was well for 3½ years. He told me that when he was diagnosed the cancer clinic had told him there was nothing that could be done and that he had a very few months left. He and his wife left the clinic beaten and depressed. When he saw me recently, he still was angry and resentful over the way they had treated him. I believe that after a patient leaves a doctor's office, he or she should feel better than when he entered. In most cases they leave their oncologist's offices feeling much worse. They appear to encourage what I have called a negative placebo reaction – the 'obecalp' reaction (placebo spelled backwards). If they are very depressed or anxious or suffer from any combination of these mood disorders, I will treat them with the appropriate medication for this.

While discussing the Measures of Life, R.M. Sapolksy refers to the investigations of two psychologists, Amos N. Tversky of Stanford University and Daniel Kahneman of the University of California at Berkeley. They investigated why people regard scenarios as unequal when in fact they are formally equivalent. He presented two scenarios. First, "You are a physician and you have a hundred sick people on your hands. If you perform treatment A, twenty people will die. If you opt for treatment B, everyone has a 20 percent chance of dying." Second, "You have a hundred sick people. If you perform treatment A, 80 people will live. If you opt for treatment B, everyone has an 80 percent chance of living." I was not surprised to learn that most people in the first scenario preferred treatment B and in the second one they preferred treatment A. As Sapolsky pointed out, "The two scenarios are formally identical; they are merely framed differently. But it turns out that for the first scenario, which states things in terms of death, people will prefer option B, whereas for the second scenario, stated in terms of survivorship, people prefer option A. When thinking about life, people prefer certainty; when thinking about death, they prefer odds, because it is always conceivable the odds can be beaten." My patients and I assume the vast majority of cancer patients prefer to bet on the odds they will survive and not on the certainty of death. The oncologists, surgeons, radiologists, and other physicians who treat these patients must take these observations to heart.

Orthomolecular treatment thus improves the quality of life. It also decreases the side effects of radiation and chemotherapy. The program is palatable. The only patients who could not follow it were those who were getting chemotherapy and suffered severe nausea and vomiting or patients who could not swallow because of lesions in their throat. Orthomolecular therapy provides a step forward in the battle against cancer which must be fully explored. There can be no logical reason today why most of the research funds should go only toward the examination of more chemotherapy and more ways of giving radiation. There must be a major expansion into the use of orthomolecular therapy to sort out the variables and to determine how to improve the therapeutic outcome of treatment.

– Abram Hoffer

Conclusions

The following conclusions were derived from the treatment and follow-up study of 134 patients in my care over almost 20 years.

1. The survival trends which appeared in the first reports I made with Dr Pauling are reconfirmed in this study. From 101 on the program, a core of 34 patients remain who have survived more than 5 years and from which 17 have survived more than 10 years. Over half of the seven who died in 1992 died of physical factors not directly related to their cancer. It is likely further deaths will increasingly come from other causes.

2. This conclusion applies only to patients who have received a combination of all the standard modalities of treatment with orthomolecular treatment.

3. Better results were found with patients who were placed on the combination soon after they were diagnosed and standard treatment was started.

4. Arbitrarily, I have concluded that there must be a minimum two-month period on the nutritional program before it can begin to demonstrate its power to prolong life. More study will be required to determine what is the minimum period.

5. Orthomolecular treatment improves the quality of life. It also decreases the side effects of radiation and chemotherapy.

6. The program is palatable. The only patients who could not follow it were those who were getting chemotherapy and suffered severe nausea and vomiting or patients who could not swallow because of lesions in their throat.

7. Orthomolecular therapy provides a step forward in the battle against cancer which must be fully explored. There can be no logical reason today why most of the research funds should go toward the examination of more chemotherapy and more ways of giving radiation. There must be a major expansion into the use of orthomolecular therapy to sort out the variables and to determine how to improve the therapeutic outcome of treatment. Enterprising medical schools should establish chairs in Orthomolecular Oncology, perhaps called the Linus Pauling Chair of Orthomolecular Oncology.

These conclusions are further substantiated by the case histories of patients recorded in the next chapter.

Of all the patients whose histories are recorded here, as of July 1999, the following have died: Numbers 84 on 2/19/99, 158 on 4/16/98, 175 on 6/26/98,

197 on 5/7/98, 201 on 7/23/97 and 250 on 5/17/97. These few deaths do not alter the conclusions drawn from the entire series of patients recorded and described in this report. I do not know the cause of death. Patient # 84, my first cancer of the pancreas patient, survived over 20 years after she was first diagnosed. I thank her for having altered my orthomolecular psychiatric practice to include the new orthomolecular oncology.

– Abram Hoffer

4 CASE HISTORIES

Preface

From the over 200 different kinds of cancer, the majority of patients in our studies suffered from the most common types, namely lung cancer, colon and rectum cancer, breast cancer, kidney and bladder cancer, prostate cancer, and leukemia. Table 12 shows the annual number of new cases of each kind of cancer diagnosed as well as the annual death and 5-year survival rates from these cancers, extrapolated from 1990 figures in the United States.

Table 13 shows the distribution of the four most common forms of cancer diagnosed among men and women in the Canadian population, extrapolated from 1996 figures.

These cancers vary in their degree of malignancy and response to conventional therapy. However, patients with all kinds of cancer have been found to benefit from orthomolecular treatment to some extent, often strikingly, either as an adjunct to appropriate conventional therapy, or alone when no effective conventional therapy is known or when the patient has reached the stage of untreatability by conventional therapy.

The following case histories of patients in our studies are prefaced by brief descriptions of the nature of these forms of cancer based on the

TABLE 12

Common Kinds of Cancer: Diagnosis, Death, and Survival Rates

	Annual number of new cases	Annual number deaths	Approximate Survival fraction
1. Lung	120,000	110,000	8%
2. Colon and rectum	120,000	60,000	50%
3. Breast	110,000	40,000	65%
4. Prostate	70,000	25,000	65%
5. Lymphomas	40,000	25,000	40%
6. Kidney and bladder	55,000	20,000	65%
7. Leukemia	25,000	10,000	60%

TABLE 13

New Cases of Cancer in Canada for 1996

	Male		Female	
	Total	Percent	Total	Percent
All	66,400		59,000	
Lung	12,616	19	7,080	12
Breast			17,700	30
Prostate	15,936	24		
Colon and rectum	8,632	13	7,670	13

descriptions provided by Dr Ewan Cameron in *Cancer and Vitamin C*, followed by a discussion of survival rates. In providing these case histories, we trust that physicians will see in the course of the patient's recovery or prolonged survival reason to use orthomolecular treatment with their own patients and that other patients will find in these cases histories of fellow patients new hope for overcoming cancer.

– Linus Pauling & Abram Hoffer

Lung Cancer

Summary

The principal cause of lung cancer is cigarette smoking. It is more common in cities than in rural areas and in cold, damp climates than in warmer and drier climates. Inhalation of industrial dust, especially dust containing asbestos fibers, is another factor. Not smoking cigarettes or breathing air contaminated with cigarette smoke is the best way to prevent lung cancer. Taking optimum amounts of vitamins may add an equal amount of protection.

Fifty years ago the disease was predominately a male disease. Now, as fewer men and more women smoke, about as many women as men contract cancer of the lung. Non-smoking wives of smokers have a higher incidence than non-smoking wives of non-smokers.

After detection of a malignant tumor in the lung, surgical treatment (removal of a lobe or an entire lung) is a valuable therapy, sometimes leading to cure. Often, however, the location of the tumor is such that operation is not possible, and often metastases have occurred, making the prognosis poor.

The use of megavitamins and other health measures is sometimes successful. The evidence so far available suggests, however, that these measures are somewhat less effective for lung cancer than for other cancers.

– Linus Pauling

In Canada, in 1996, 33 out of every 100,000 females will die from lung cancer, 4 times the 1969 rate. Nine out of 10 are caused by smoking. Men still have a higher rate of lung cancer, but it is getting lower and is rising for women. Out of 66,400 cases of male cancer, lung cancer will account for 19 percent. It accounts for the highest proportion of deaths from all cancer, 33 percent in men, and in women 21 percent. The survival rates of the lung patients I saw is shown in Table 14.

– Abram Hoffer

TABLE 14
The Survival By Years of All Lung Cancer Patients on the Vitamin Regimen and on Standard Treatment Only, Seen Between 1978 and the end of 1994.

On Orthomolecular Plus Standard Treatment					Standard Only		
Year could have lived	Years at risk	Number at end of year could have lived	Alive alive	Percent	N	Alive	%
		1994	1	63	23	37	
1993	2	54	11	20			
1992	3	40	7	18			
1991	4	35	4	11	Eighteen controls died the first year.		
1990	5	29	2	7			
1989	6	21	2	10			
1988	7	14	1	14			
1987	8	10	1	10			
1986	9	—	—	—			
1985	10	—	—	—			
1978 to 1984		8	1	14			

Survival Rates

The first column is the year showing the total number of patients seen. The second column shows the number of years they could all have lived. The third column shows the number of patients, the fourth column shows the number reaching that survival period. Thus of the patients seen by 1990 only two survived five years.

Out of 31 female patients, 16 lived one year, 10 lived 2 years, 7 lived 3 years, 4 lived 4 years, and 2 lived 7 years. Eight are still alive. Out of 32 male patients, 9 lived one year, 1 died the second year, and 1 the third year.

Between 1 January 1980 and the end of 1995, I saw 93 patients with cancer of the lung. The number alive and dead for each of five follow up years is shown in Table 15. Seven patients lived for 4 or more years.

TABLE 15 Lung Cancer Survivors							
Years Following First Visit		Alive					
Seen by year end	Number Seen	Number Alive					Percent
		1	2	3	4	5	
1990	28					2	9
1991	35				4		11
1992	48			7			15
1993	54		11				28
1994	63	23					37

Case Histories

(1) Case #1

Born in 1920, she was first seen in April 1984. On 2 November 1983 she had suffered terrible flu, a cold, a cough for four months with increasing amounts of sputum, weight loss and lethargy. On examination there was reduced air entry into the right upper lobe and dullness to percussion. The X-ray revealed collapse of the right upper lobe. A mass was felt during mediastinoscopy and fluid was aspirated containing pus. The surgeon thought it was a bronchiogenic carcinoma that had broken down. Later the surgeon saw a tumor on the right side which had totally occluded the right upper bronchus and had extended to the lateral wall of the right main bronchus and to a level below the carina. The pathological report showed a poorly differentiated squamous cell carcinoma. This was considered non-resectable because it was unlikely she would tolerate the procedure. Her prognosis was considered poor because the tumor would probably not resolve completely and the possibility of distant metastases was high. She was told she could expect to live about one year.

On 3 January 1984 she started to receive cobalt irradiation until 14 February 1984, receiving 20 sessions. A month later she had an upper respiratory infection and was given antibiotics. On 24 April 1984 she was started on the vitamin regimen including vitamin C 12 g, niacinamide 1.5 g, zinc sulfate 220 mg, vitamin E 800 IU, selenium 200 micrograms and a multimineral preparation.

In March 1986 she complained of intermittent claudication. She was high in cholesterol and one artery was clogged in her right leg. I added inositol niacinate 1.5 g, calcium 1,000 mg, and magnesium 500 mg. A month later she was able to walk four blocks. In January 1993 she had a mild stroke, so mild that after intensive investigation in hospital the diagnosis still was uncertain, but she was left with mild speech impairment which cleared in a few months. On 24 December 1993, there was no recurrence of her cancer but both legs were badly swollen and she was waiting for a bed for investigation. Her mood had been good until this had happened over the past few weeks. Later in December 1993 she suffered a stroke which left her speech impaired. After that she had three episodes of flu. She died 25 January 1994 at age 73 just three months before her tenth anniversary of having first seen me.

(2) Case #37

Born in 1927, she was first seen in March 1981. In December 1980 she had experienced sharp right-sided chest pain. An x-ray showed a large mass in her right lung. A bronchoscope in December 1980 showed a visible tumor involving the lateral wall of the right lower lobe bronchus and extending into the right upper lobe bronchus and occluding the oriface of the superior segment of the right lower lobe. She had a small oat cell bronchiogenic carcinoma. She also had an ill-defined area in the left tempero partietal region. She was considered inoperable and she was given radiotherapy to her brain starting in January 1981, and chemotherapy which was completed in June 1981. This was then followed by radiotherapy to the right lung completed in July 1981. A note in the cancer clinic report states, "This lady elected to go ahead with chemotherapy. She understands it's palliative and not curative."

On 4 March 1981 I advised her to take ascorbic acid 12 g, niacinamide 1.5 g, a B complex preparation containing zinc. At the end of 11 years there has been no recurrence. Her memory is very poor, probably due to the radiation to her head. She was on the total vitamin program probably not more than one year. March 1992 she was well and was taken off the follow up program. She was still well in October 1996.

(3) Case #97

Born in 1933, she was first seen in September 1987. The middle and lower right lung had been removed in August 1985. She came to see me depressed and concerned about a recurrence. Her depression was being treated with an amine oxidase inhibitor, which she thought could have been a factor in the development of her cancer. I advised her that this was unlikely and to start the following vitamin program: ascorbic acid 4 grams t.i.d., niacin 500 mg t.i.d., folic acid 5 mg b.i.d., B-complex 50s t.i.d., zinc gluconate 50 mg od, and selenium 0.200 mg b.i.d. On 31 December 1989 she was well and following the program, except for the niacin. She had flushed too much on niacin and had reduced the dose to 250 mg b.i.d.. She died 1 November 1990.

(4) Case #183

Born in 1916, she was first seen in October 1990. Early in 1990 this patient developed a lump in a left neck gland. At biopsy on 1 May 1990, an adeno-carcinoma was found but there was no primary. In June the tumor was resected, but because of its proximity to the jugular vein could not be entirely removed. Following that she received 10 radiation sessions over a two-week period, and she was on tamoxifen. About the same time she started herself on a vitamin program which she had been following for three months before I saw her, and she felt a lot better. She had been taking vitamins for many years. She had a second lump develop on the right side of her neck but it had stopped growing and may have started to recede, as had some post-radiation nodules. She had a cough she found troublesome which she thought might be due to allergies. On her own she had been taking: germanium 150 ug od, vitamin A and D containing 10,000 IU of A, evening primrose oil 1 gram per day, EPA 1 gram per day, vitamin E 400 IU per day, beta carotene 10,000 IU t.i.d., coenzyme Q_{10} 30 mg per day, a super mineral preparation, B-complex 75 mg od, B-6 125 mg od, quercetin 1 gram per day, selenium 200 mcg t.i.d., zinc citrate 50 mg od, vitamin C 24 grams per day. I modified her program only slightly, changing her beta carotene to 25,000 IU per day, the selenium to 200 mcg b.i.d., and adding aspirin 325 mg od.

On 3 December 1990, she reported all the lumps in her skin were gone. In April 1991 her daughter reported that her mother had been in hospital in Hawaii for seven days after developing fluid in her chest and abdominal cavity. The fluid was drained. A primary was discovered in the lower lobe of her left lung. In hospital for one month a lot of fluid was drained from her abdomen and chest. She had been given antibiotics and 35 radiation treatments to her chest and neck but had been off her vitamin program. After discharge, she resumed her nutrient intake. By July her strength was returning, her appetite was okay, and her weight was steady.

Late in November 1991 she reported she was better, but that she needed afternoon naps or she tired. She was able to tolerate ascorbic acid 16 grams per day. Her last CT scan was clear, she had no surface lumps, but had a tiny nodule on her neck. Her mood was good, she was very cheerful and felt really good. In September 1992 she still coughed and had some sputum, but she was otherwise well. In November 1992 she was still well and was on her program. Again on 23 November 1993 she was well. In April 1992 two nodes of cancer were found in her chest. She received more radiation and since then has been well. Her mood was good and she was optimistic. She was still on the entire program. On 15 December 1993 she increased the coenzyme Q_{10} to 240 mg daily.

On 22 March 1994, she was in hospital. She had become short of breath. One liter of fluid was removed. After this was done she was found to have two lesions in her left lung. She was to receive more radiation. Her mood was good. While in hospital she remained on her nutrient program. She died 24 June 1994.

(5) Case #324

Born in 1929, she was first seen in July 1991. In August 1990 she began to cough. On examination she had a large lesion, the size of a large orange, in her right lung which was attached to bone. She was given 20 radiation treatments which shrank the tumor. Three months before I saw her she developed pain in her back from a hairline fracture. The last x-ray examination before I saw her showed the tumor had regressed. I advised her to take ascorbic acid 12 g, niacinamide 1.5 g, B complex-50, folic acid 10 mg, vitamin E 1200 IU, selenium 1000 mcg, beta carotene 100,000 IU, boron 3 mg, and manganese 15 mg, all daily. On December 31 she reported her x-ray at the end of October showed no tumor, only some scar tissue. She was able to take 9 grams of vitamin C and had decreased the amount of some of the other vitamins and minerals. In July 1992 she had occasional back pain and was still on the program. She was alive in July 1996.

(6) Case #351

Born in 1932, she was first seen in June 1991. In May 1991 she suffered the flu and cough. On routine x-ray a shadow was observed in her lung which had apparently been there one year before. A biopsy was positive. At first she refused to have surgery but later agreed to it in July. Three years earlier she had a myocardial infarct, later angina, and in January 1989 she had angioplasty. She had started to take vitamin C 6 grams per day, coenzyme Q_{10} 200 mg, and beta carotene. I advised her to increase the vitamin C to 12 g, to add niacin 1.5 g, B complex-50, beta carotene 75,000 IU, vitamin E 800 IU, selenium 600 mcg, zinc citrate 50 mg, and folic acid 10 mg, all daily. On 11 June 1992 she was well and felt good. On 22 February 1994 she was getting on well. Again in June 1996 she was well.

(7) Case #429

Born in 1943, she was first seen March 1992. In 1974 she had a radical mastectomy followed by 15 sessions of irradiation. About mid-1988 a lesion was found in her right lung and the middle lobe was removed. Two years later it recurred but was very slow growing. I advised her to take ascorbic acid 12 g, niacinamide 2.0 g, B complex 50, selenium 600 mcg, beta carotene 50,000 IU, vitamin E 800 IU, and zinc citrate 50 mg. On 31 December 1992 she was well and was on the full program.

In March 1994 she discovered cervical nodes, and on 16 March 1995 she was very ill. Her tumor in her lung was enlarging rapidly. She had more radiation. Medication given caused perforation of her intestine. She had lost 40 pounds and was no longer able to follow the regimen. She died 17 March 1995.

– Abram Hoffer

Colon and Rectum Cancer

Summary

Cancers of the colon and rectum kill about 60,000 people each year in the United States. It is likely that most of these cancers are caused by carcinogenic substances in the feces and that a large decrease in incidence could be achieved by destroying these substances or by decreasing the exposure of the intestinal wall to them. In 1979 it was shown by workers in the Ludwig Cancer Institute in Toronto, Canada, that a high intake of vitamin C destroys the mutagens, which often act as carcinogens, in human feces. Moreover, constipation, which increases the length of time of exposure of the walls of the colon and rectum to the carcinogens, increases the probability of developing cancer of the lower bowel. It is thus important to avoid constipation and thereby decrease the length of time that the waste products of digestion remaining the lower bowel.

One way of doing this is to take regularly enough vitamin C or enough fruit to have a significant laxative action. Another way is to eat a high-fiber diet. The high-fiber diet increases the bulk of the waste material enough to cause the bowels to move it along more rapidly and also to dilute the carcinogens, thus further decreasing the exposure of the walls of the colon and rectum to them.

We estimate that following one or another of these practices would decrease the incidence of these cancers by more than 50 percent. Part of the basis for this estimate is that cancer of the lower bowel is far less common in primitive societies than in the Western world. In the less developed countries, the diets contain far more roughage than in the United States and Europe. It is also interesting that among primitive societies cancer of the small intestine is rare, causing only about 2 percent as many deaths as cancer of the colon and rectum. This fact may be explained by the relatively rapid movement of the waste material along the small intestine.

There are some other predisposing factors to cancers of the lower bowel. One is the inherited tendency to develop colonic polyps (multiple benign colonic tumors). People with this trait are almost certain ultimately to develop cancer of the colon if the occurrence of the polyps is not prevented by regular high doses of vitamin C. Also, some patients with ulcerative colitis that remains uncontrolled for ten years or more frequently succumb to colonic cancer.

Cancer of the colon is usually recognized through anemia from blood loss or loss in body weight caused by toxic substances released by the ulcerated tumor. Cancer of the rectum leads to bowel irregularity, blood in the feces, a constant urge to defecate, and a feeling of incomplete bowel evacuation. Signs like these should be immediately brought to the attention of the physician. Early identification, before the formation of metastases, which often occur in the liver, is very important. Early surgery can lead to cure. Postoperative radiotherapy has no value for colonic cancer, but may be helpful for cancer of the rectum. At present, it is generally accepted that chemotherapy has no overall value for these cancers; the debilitating and unpleasant effects of the toxicity of the chemotherapeutic agents are more than enough to negate the small increase in survival time experienced by a small fraction of the patients given courses of chemotherapy. Vitamin C and the other factors in the regimen described in this book are, however, of great value.

– Linus Pauling

In Canada, out of over 60,0000 cases of male cancers, cancer of the colon and rectum accounts for 13 percent. Out of almost 60,000 cases of female cancer, it accounts for in 13 percent as well.

The survival rates for all colorectals cancers I have seen are shown in Table 16.

– Abram Hoffer

Survival Rates

The survival was the same for both male and female patients. Only 2 patients out of 13 not on treatment survived one year. This is consistent with the published data for these cancers already well established and no longer stageable or treatable. The 5 to 10 year survival for the treated group was much better, about 40 percent.

By the end of 1995 I had seen 62 patients with colon cancer and 3 with cancer of the rectum. Of the 65, 51 were treated and 14 were control. The follow up data is shown in Table 17.

TABLE 16
The Survival By Years of All Colorectal Cancer Patients on the Vitamin Regimen and on Standard Treatment Only, Seen Between 1978 and the end of 1993.

On Orthomolecular Plus Standard Treatment					Standard Only
Year Seen have lived	Years could risk	Number at of year	Alive at end	Percent alive	
1994	1	47	33	70	Out of 13 control patients 11 died the first year, 2 died the second year.
1993	2	38	27	71	
1992	3	36	21	58	
1991	4	26	11	42	
1990	5	24	7	29	
1989	6	16	6	38	
1988	7	12	4	33	
1987	8	10	4	40	
1986	9	7	3	43	
1985	10	5	2	40	
1978 to 1984	11	4	1	25	

Case Histories

(of patients alive five years or more)

(1) Case #15

Born in 1927, he was first seen in December 1985. In 1978 he had begun to suffer abdominal pain and constipation from diverticulosis. He hemorrhaged in December 1986. He came to see me first in April 1985 complaining of severe anxiety and tension. His whole body was rigid from tension as if he was surrounded by body armor. I modified his diet to remove all free sugars and added ascorbic acid 1 g t.i.d., niacin 1 g t.i.d., vitamin E 400 iu b.i.d., zinc sulfate 220 mg od, and dolomite 2 tablets t.i.d. He also came to see me regularly for psychotherapy. On 19 December 1986 carcinoma of the colon above the transverse and sigmoid area was diagnosed. The tumor and some of the colon was removed. I increased his

TABLE 17
Colon Cancer Survivors

On Regimen		N	Years following first visit 1	2	3	4	5	Percent Dec. 31/95
Yes —	Alive	51	39	31	27	25	25	49
	Died		12	8	4	2	0	
	Total dead		20	24	26	26		
No —	Alive	15	2	0				0
	Dead		13	2				

ascorbic acid to 12 g daily and added 500 mcg of selenium. In February 1987, no tumor was evident on colonoscopic examination and there were no polyps. He was free of anxiety. He then stopped taking the nutrients. In July 1987 he became constipated and again began to follow the regimen, increasing his ascorbic acid to 25 g daily. On 28 March 1988 he was well; on 31 December 31 1995 he was alive and well and was free of anxiety, tension, or depression.

His wife, Case # 677, born in 1936, was found to have cancer of the ovaries. A large ovarian growth was removed in September 1995. They then went to New York, where she had relatives, and attended Dr N. Gonzalez. She was very concerned because she thought the cancer had been moving very quickly from a time late last January when nothing could be felt until the present when a large size tumor was discovered. She refused to accept chemotherapy. Her husband remained well during this very difficult period. In the fall of 1996 she suffered a recurrence but is still receiving complementary therapy.

(2) Case #87

Born in 1952, he was first seen in April 1982. Early in 1981 he suffered stomach problems with some rectal bleeding. In December 1981 he was discovered to have cancer of his colon, the transverse section, which was resected. The tumor had perforated the bowel and was infected. Some of his spleen was removed, but there had been no spread. I advised him to take ascorbic acid 12 g, B-complex-100, vitamin E 400 iu, selenium 400 mcg, zinc sulfate

220 mg, and calcium magnesium 6 tablets, all daily. In April 1988 his spleen had regenerated. On 23 October 1992 he was normal and on minor vitamin supplements. After 11 years he was still well and was removed from our follow-up list.

(3) Case #95

Born in 1922, she was first seen in July 1981. In 1971 a large fibroma had been removed. In 1973 she suffered from repeated hemorrhages with her periods. In 1977 she had a small stroke which left her for a long time with right-sided weakness and her thinking was fuzzy. She had suffered a lot of family stress. She was divorced from a schizophrenic husband and lived with her brutal addicted son who, a few days after I saw her, blackened her eye. I advised her to start on niacin 1.5 g, ascorbic acid 1.5 g, and zinc gluconate 100 mg and discussed her relationship to her son. On 24 September she was better and stronger.

However, in October 1982 she had again been injured by her son. I increased her niacin to 2 g, adding pyridoxine 100 mg and folic acid 5 mg. In December 1982 she was again much better. On 12 December 1983 she told me her son had at last moved away. She was very weak. In February 1984 she was depressed, but it was not as severe as her depression the year before.In May 1985 she had trouble with her vision from cataracts and they were removed.

In October 1986 she was found to have cancer of the bowel which was resected. I increased her ascorbic acid to 12 g, changed niacin to inositol niacinate 1.5 g, and added selenium 400 mcg. In December 1986 she required further abdominal surgery to repair some damage. There was no evidence of recurrence. In May 1989 the cancer had occluded her bowel. This was resected and she was left with a colostomy.

On 22 November 1990 she told me she had not been able to follow the full program. I advised her to take ascorbic acid 8 g, niacin 2 g, selenium 400 mcg, vitamin E 800 iu, and Q_{10} 90 mg, daily. I doubt she was able to follow this program. She developed congestive heart failure and was given digoxin but was not able to follow the correct dose. She died 11 August 1992. The coroner concluded she died from congestive heart failure. She had excessive amounts of digoxin in her blood. At autopsy she was found to have adeno carcinoma of the peritoneum with a left hydronephrosis. The cancer had recurred but she did not die from it.

(4) Case #146

Born 1917, she was first seen in April 12 1989. In July 1986 one foot of the transverse colon was resected. There was by then some extension into her liver. Before the operation, there had been few if any symptoms but it was detected on physical examination. Soon after she placed herself on a moderate-dose vitamin program, including 1750 mg of vitamin C daily. She came to see me because she was concerned whether this program was adequate. I suggested since there was no evidence of recurrence that she follow the program with a few changes as follows: vitamin C 1750 mg od, niacin 0.5 g t.i.d., selenium 200 mcg b.i.d., B-complex 50 mg od.

One month later she found that she could not tolerate the niacin flush, so the niacin was replaced with niacinamide 0.5 g t.i.d. On 7 January 1992 she was normal and her mood was good. She was still on the same program. On 17 May 1993 she was well, even though she was not following the program and had forgotten what vitamins she had been taking before. In April 1996 she was again well.

(5) Case #157

Born 1939, she was first seen in October 1990. In May 1990 this patient noticed some blood in her stool, but nothing positive was found. She went to Europe in mid-July and developed bladder pain. On return home, investigation, including barium enema, revealed cancer of the colon. Some of her bladder was removed; there was no extension into it. The colon was resected and 4 out of 18 nodes were positive, but apparently there were no other metastases. She started on chemotherapy, having a very severe reaction to the first one: her white blood count went down to 30 and her neutrophils to 16. After that they did go up, but it was necessary to watch the chemotherapy very carefully. It was considered unusual to react badly to that type of chemotherapy. After the last session before she was seen here, she developed a high fever.

Before she was diagnosed with cancer she had been very healthy, except that she had been constipated for several years, requiring constant treatment with Agarol, a laxative. She was very physically fit and was active in sports.

She was started on the following: ascorbic acid 4 grams t.i.d., Niacinamide 500 mg t.i.d., B-complex 50s od, vitamin E 400 iu b.i.d., cod liver oil 2 capsules per day, beta carotene 25,000 iu t.i.d., vitamin K 5 mg od, selenium 200 mcg t.i.d., cal/mag 3 tablets per day, magnesium oxide 420 mg per day, and zinc citrate 50 mg per day.

She telephoned in November 1990. She was on calcium ascorbate 6 grams per day, having been told by someone she did not require more. I asked her to increase it back up to 12 grams per day. She was no longer constipated, her mood was good, and she planned to discontinue chemotherapy. December 1990 she felt great, had no problems, was not constipated, and felt normal. She telephoned in March 1991 to state she had been skiing and developed diarrhea at 7,000 ft elevation but not at the lower levels. She had a lot of energy, but occasionally got short of breath, which could come at any time. She was still on chemotherapy. On 12 February 1992 she reported she was normal. There was no sign of cancer at her last check up, and she was following the full program. She was very cheerful. In October 1996 she was well.

(6) Case #255

Born 1934, she was first seen in July 1985. In December 1984, cancer had been resected from her sigmoid colon. Out of 7 glands, one had metastases. Then she was given 20 radiation sessions. In addition she had been depressed following a series of marital problems, for which she was receiving psychotherapy. I advised her to stay on her diet, which consisted mostly of ensure mixed with yogurt, but to add one new food each week as a test of her tolerance. She also was advised to take ascorbic acid 12 grams daily, niacinamide 500 mg t.i.d., B-complex (100) od, selenium 400 mcg daily, zinc gluconate 50 mg od, and calcium and magnesium tablets 4 daily. I gave her mycostatin for yeast infection. One month later she reported she could only take 1.5 grams of vitamin C daily because of severe diarrhea. She was able to tolerate the rest of the program. She felt much better and was not as confused as she had been.

On 24 June 1992 she was normal. This was reported to me by her son whom she had sent to me for treatment. She was still following the vitamin program. In December 1996 she was well. Her three last sigmnoidoscopic examinations were normal.

(7) Case #302

Born in 1917, she was first seen in November 1987. Eight years before I saw her she was given a colostomy for colon cancer. In 1984 she suffered from a bleeding ulcer. Apart from a few other complaints unrelated to her colostomy, she got on well but she was concerned about a possible recurrence and came for advice. I suggested she follow the following program: ascorbic acid 3 g, niacin 1.5 g, B-complex (50), selenium 200 mcg, vitamin E 400 iu, and calcium magnesium two tablets, all daily. She was seen several times, the last in February 1992 for other problems. On 10 November 1992 she was free of cancer and was still on the program.

On 13 December 1993 she told me she had had an hysterectomy one month earlier because a small tumor was found, Stage 2, after her second d & c. It had apparently not spread. She was depressed over this second assault on her by the cancer, yet her colon remained normal. I increased her ascorbic acid to 6 g, increased her folic acid to 15 mg, and added Q_{10} 150 mg daily. For her depression I added an antidepressant. On 10 February 1994 she reported she had one long radiation session to her abdomen. I have continued her on an antidepressant and added Q_{10} 300 mg daily in October 1996.

– Abram Hoffer

Breast Cancer

Summary

For many years cancer of the breast was the principal cause of death of women by cancer, but, without having been significantly decreased, it has now been passed by cancer of the lung because of the increased tendency of women to smoke cigarettes. We may hope that women will soon begin to follow the example of men, who now smoke much less that 40 years ago. Cigarette smoking not only causes lung cancer, but also increases the death rate by other diseases – heart disease, infectious diseases, diabetes, and other kinds of cancer, including breast cancer. A woman who regularly smokes cigarettes at the rate of one pack a day has twice the chance of dying of breast cancer as a woman who does not smoke.

Hormonal factors are also involved in breast cancer. This disease occurs more often in unmarried women than in married women, and least often in women who have breast fed a number of children.

Diagnosis is made by the discovery of a painless lump in the breast, with later dimpling of the overlying skin and retraction of the nipple. Metastases occur to the lymphatic nodes in the armpits and chest wall, and later to the bones and the lung.

Surgical treatment, a simple lumpectomy or removal of the breast and involved lymph nodes, is often successful. Extensive and crippling surgery (the Halsted procedure) is now rarely carried out. As with many other kinds of cancer, the orthomolecular regimen described in this book has great value.

Chemotherapy has little value in the treatment of breast cancer, although oncologists continue to administer new combinations of chemotherapeutic drugs to breast cancer patients in the effort to find a useful therapy. A few years ago the National Cancer Institute announced that chemotherapy had considerable value for younger breast cancer patients, but much less for older (post menopausal) patients. Members of Congress asked that this question be studied, and a comparison was made of the survival times of women who had developed breast cancer when not over age 45 years and who had received chemotherapy with those who had not received chemotherapy. This study showed little difference in the survival times of the two groups. The prepared report had the title "Chemotherapy Found Not To Be Effective Against Breast Cancer in Premenopausal Women." The National Cancer Institute objected to this title and to some of the statements in the report. The title was then changed to "A Study of the Value of Chemotherapy in the Treatment of Breast Cancer in Premenopausal Women," and some of the statements in the first draft were omitted or revised. This report supports the opinion that at the present time chemotherapy has not been shown to have value in the treatment of breast cancer in younger women.

– Linus Pauling

In Canada, about 30 percent of female cancers are breast cancers and it causes 21 percent of the deaths. The incidence is increasing, mostly among women over age 60. In 1995, 103 of every 100,000 women were diagnosed, up from 78 in 1969.

In our studies, the long term extension of life for every type of cancer was significantly better with the addition of orthomolecular treatment. But patients with some types of cancer responded better than did other groups. To compare these different classes of patients, I will compare the ten-year follow-up data where there is a reasonable number of patients per group. The standard will be the overall response rate, which was about 40 percent recovery for the last five years of the ten year follow-up period. Any group with a better survival rate than the standard obviously has responded better and therefore has a better prognosis when treated with this combined approach.

This was the largest group. The survival of the orthomolecular combined with standard treatment group was much better than the survival of the group receiving only standard treatment. As with the total, group survival was around 40 percent after eight years but then fell off over the next two years. However, there were few patients in the group who could have lived for ten years. Over the next five years a better estimate of the overall ten-year survival rate will be available. The survival data is given in Table 18.

Survival Rates

Age was a factor in the breast cancer group. Out of 24 born before 1930, 21 percent lived 10 years. From the group born later than that, out of 22, 64 percent lived ten years.

Between January 1980 and the end of April 1996, I saw 198 patients with breast cancer. Table 19 shows the number of patients who lived by year and the number alive today. These patients were given standard modern treatment including surgery, chemotherapy, radiation, and all the combinations of these three.

During the five years ending with 1995, I had seen 153 patients with breast cancer. Their five year survival is shown below as well. Of 68 patients seen by the end of 1990 who could have survived five years, only 36 or 53 percent did. Of 118 seen by the end of 1992 who could have survived 3 years, only 66 or 56 percent did.

Comparing patients who died within one year of having been seen and those who lived at least five years, 21 patients out of 184 who were the megavitamin regimen died in the first year and the average time between the onset of symptoms of their disease and when they were seen was 3.3

TABLE 18

The Survival By Years of All Breast Cancer Patients on the Vitamin Regimen and on Standard Treatment Only Seen Between 1978 and the end of 1993.

On Orthomolecular Plus Standard Treatment					Standard Only
Year Seen	Years could have lived	Number at risk	Alive at end of year	Percent alive	
1994	1	154	134	87	
1993	2	130	89	68	Out of 14 in the
1992	3	111	67	61	non treated group
1991	4	69	42	61	10 died in the
1990	5	51	27	53	first year, 2 in
1989	6	39	21	54	the second year.
1988	7	29	13	45	One is alive
1987	8	22	10	45	5 years, the
1986	9	16	5	31	other 4 years.
1985	10	12	3	25	

years. They were almost entirely grade three and four, most of them having relapsed from previous treatment. There were 36 alive for at least five years. The interval between their first symptoms and when I first saw them was 1.3 years. From the control group 11 out of 14 died the first year and two survived five years.

Survival from breast cancer is a function of the involvement of the rest of the body. As it spreads into nodes and to other parts of the body, survival becomes more difficult. The grading of breast cancer is based upon this. I have therefore examined the relationship between survival and whether or not lymph nodes have been involved and whether or not there has been further spread, i.e., metastasis. This is shown in Tables 20a-d.

As would be expected, the best outcome was achieved by patients whose cancer had not spread. About 80 percent were well after 5 years. Based upon the entire cancer series so far, this predicts that these patients will survive at least 15 years after their first attack by the cancer. About 80 per-

TABLE 19 Breast Cancer Survivors, Percent							
Years following first visit		Alive					
Seen by year end	Number Seen	Number Alive					Percent
		1	2	3	4	5	
1990	68					36	53
1991	87				52		60
1992	118			66			56
1993	129		129				68
1994	153	133					87

cent of women with breast cancer which has not spread will achieve a 15-year cure rate – i.e., they will be cured. The next best outcome group are patients with positive nodes but no further metastasis. About 50 percent will reach a five year cure rate, estimated to reach 15 years. The next two groups – i.e., patients with metastasis, whether or not they have nodal involvement – have about the same prognosis. About 35 percent will reach an estimated 15-year cure rate. This is shown in Figure 5.

Patients without node involvement had a better prognosis. From the whole group, 25 patients had no node involvement. Their mean survival to now is 3.5 years. Twenty-two had 1 to 3 nodes and their mean survival is 2.9 years, while 92 had 4 to 12 nodes and this group survived 2.3 years. In 10 patients the tumor had spread into nodes as well as into other areas. The number of nodes involved in this small group made no difference to survival.

In 37 patients with only nodes involved, there was a difference in favor of the group with the lesser number of nodes involved. Twenty-one had between 1 and 3 nodes and they have a survival of 3.1 years. Sixteen had between 4 and 12 nodes and they have survived 2.4 years.

Case Histories

For each organ attacked by the cancer, I will provide a few case histories of failures and more case histories of successful treatment. I include the

TABLE 20A

Survival of Breast Cancer Cases with No Positive Nodes and No Metastasis

Seen by year end	Number Seen	Number Alive					Percent
		1	2	3	4	5	
1990	26					20	77
1991	35				31		89
1992	45			38			84
1993	55		48				87
1994	66	61					92

TABLE 20B

Survival of Breast Cancer Cases with Positive Nodes and No Metastasis

Seen by year end	Number Seen	Number Alive					Percent
		1	2	3	4	5	
1990	16					8	50
1991	21				11		52
1992	27			17			63
1993	32		22				69
1994	42	40					95

TABLE 20C

Survival of Breast Cancer Cases with No Nodes Positive but with Metastasis

Seen by year end	Number Seen	Number Alive					Percent
		1	2	3	4	5	
1990	14					4	29
1991	19				4		21
1992	22			6			27
1993	24		11				46
1994	26	19					73

TABLE 20D
Survival of Breast Cancer Cases with Both Positive Nodes and Metastasis

Seen by year end	Number Seen	Number Alive					Percent
		1	2	3	4	5	
1990	10					4	40
1991	10				5		50
1992	14			6			43
1993	15		6				40
1994	16	11					60

failures simply to avoid leaving the impression that the treatment we recommend is the final perfect treatment. I will not include all the failures because every oncologist is familiar with failure and does not need to reminded of it any more, but reading clinical accounts of these type of successes may persuade them to try out the treatment.

Patients Who Died Within One Year After Starting Program

(1) Case #156
Born in 1939, she was first seen in July 1989. In 1978 this patient had received a modified radical mastectomy; no lymph nodes were involved. She was well until 1989 when she began to notice flashes of light in her right eye. Seven days later she developed pain in her groin and knee, especially on walking. On x-ray she was discovered to have multiple metastases to her legs, pelvis, neck, upper spine, eye, and the bones of her upper arms. A brain scan was negative. She received radiation to the secondary in her eye, receiving four sessions.

On her own she had started herself on a program including ascorbic acid 4 grams per day, pau d'arco (a herbal preparation), Coenzyme Q_{10} 30 mg t.i.d., beta carotene 25,000 iu t.i.d., germanium 25 mg t.i.d., B-complex 6 tablets per day, vitamin E 400 iu t.i.d., lecithin 1.2 grams t.i.d., zinc t.i.d. (dose unknown), calcium/magnesium t.i.d. (dose unknown), and had been on this program 6 weeks when she came to see me. She felt that as a

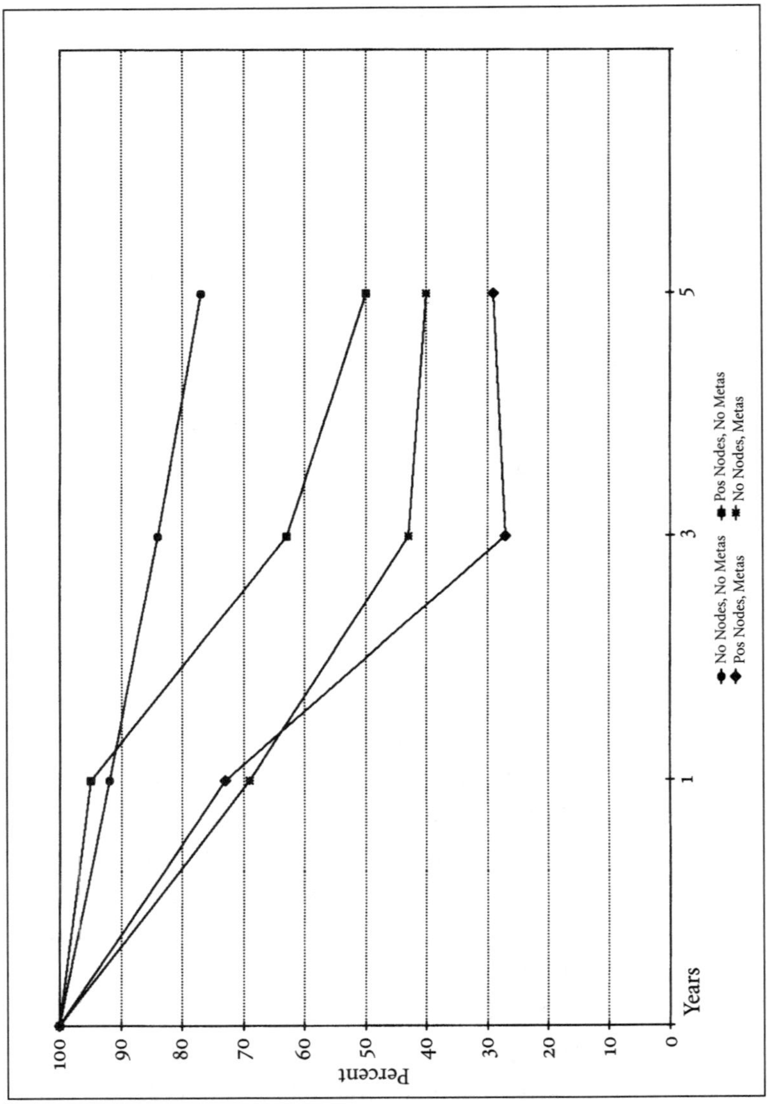

FIGURE 5
Cancer Survival, Positive Nodes and Metastis

result of this program she had much more energy; before that she was totally exhausted and wanted to stay in bed all the time.

Her program was modified to the following: ascorbic acid 2 grams t.i.d., calcium ascorbate 2 grams t.i.d., niacinamide 500 mg t.i.d., B-complex 50s od, coenzyme Q_{10} 30 mg t.i.d., beta carotene 25,000 iu od, germanium 25 mg t.i.d., vitamin E 400 iu t.i.d., lecithin 1.2 grams t.i.d., zinc t.i.d., calcium/magnesium t.i.d., linseed oil 3 tbsp per day, selenium 200 mcg t.i.d., Slow-K 600 mg t.i.d.

She died 19 February 1990, 8 months after I first saw her. The quality of her life was improved by the treatment, however.

(2) Case #430

Born 1952, she was first seen in August 1992. In June 1990 she had a partial mastectomy, followed by 15 radiation treatments. She also had 4 sessions of chemotherapy. One year later it recurred on the same side. In June and July she had respiratory symptoms. She was given more radiation and more chemotherapy. There were masses in both lungs but her bones were clear. When I first saw her, she was very short of breath and needed a portable oxygen tank with her. I advised her to take ascorbic acid 12 g, niacinamide 3 g, B-complex 50, beta carotene 100,000 iu, selenium 600 mcg, and zinc sulfate 100 mg, all daily. Her blood copper and zinc levels were 127 and 92, respectively, ratio 1.38. She was given additional different chemotherapy and required transfusions. On 21 September 1992 she appeared to be improving. She died 28 October 28 1992, two months after I saw her.

(3) Case #486

Born in 1930, she was first seen in May 1993. In fall 1988 she had a lumpectomy followed by 28 radiations treatments. All the glands were negative. One year later a secondary was removed, followed by 20 more radiation sessions. She tried tamoxifen for five months and had to discontinue. She noted a lump below the right side of her neck which later became more noticeable as a swelling. She also had several small lesions in her lungs. I advised her to take ascorbic acid 12 g, niacinamide 1.5 g, folic acid 15 mg, beta carotene 50,000 iu, vitamin E 800 iu, selenium 400 mcg, and zinc citrate 50 mg, all daily. She died 18 April 1994, 11 months after I first saw her.

(4) Case #650
Born in 1926, she was first seen in April 1995. The patient had a left mastectomy in May 1986, followed by radiation, 5 treatments. Her nodes were negative. She was well until July 1992 when she was found to have metastases to both lungs and fluid at the base of the right lung. In August the fluid was drained. Biopsy reported breast cancer cells in the fluid. She was then injected with Tetracycline on the right side. Following that she had chemotherapy. In February 1993 she went into congestive heart failure. In March 1995 she broke her collar bone while she was sitting up in bed, shifting her weight backwards. She had extensive metastases to her bones, her ribs on both sides, collarbone on the right side, in her skull on the right side, and her backbone. She was to begin additional chemotherapy at the Cancer Clinic.

The patient was advised to continue her diet which was more vegetarian and low fat, low sugar. To this I added ascorbic acid 4 g t.i.d. to bowel tolerance level, folic acid 5 mg t.i.d., niacinamide 500 mg b.i.d., B-complex 50 mg od, vitamin E 400 iu b.i.d., beta carotene 25,000 iu od, zinc citrate 50 mg od, selenium 200 mcg per day, coenzyme Q_{10} 300 mg per day. She died 5 October 1995, about 6 months after I first saw her.

Patients Still Alive Five Years and More

(1) Case #135
Born in 1953, she was first seen in July 1990. During October 1989 she felt a lump in her right axilla which was cancerous. She received radiation for three weeks, two per week, and on 19 January 1990 had a lumpectomy. After that she received chemotherapy once every month for four months. She had heard Dr Linus Pauling's lecture on cancer and vitamin C and wanted to start on a proper preventive program. She was advised to take the following nutrients: ascorbic acid 4 grams t.i.d., niacinamide 0.5 g t.i.d., selenium 200 mcg b.i.d., B-complex 50s od, vitamin E 400 iu od, Chromium 200 mcg od. In July 1996 she was well.

(2) Case #158
Born in 1914, she was first seen in January 1990. This patient first came to

see me in July 1980 in the hope something could be done about the onset of sudden blindness of her right eye. She had lost vision in her left eye some twelve years earlier, again very suddenly.

When I saw her again in January 1990, she reported she had been diagnosed with breast cancer in early December 1989. She had remained on the original vitamin program only two months, not being able to follow it because of her husband's illness and eventual death two years later, and because she had been traveling and had herself also been ill. She had been legally blind for many years but still lived alone with home help, was independent, and was able to get around.

Surgery, radiation, and chemotherapy had been recommended for her, but she was opposed to any standard treatment. She had no pain. She had started on Essiac and was on vitamin C 4 grams per day. I recommended the following program: ascorbic acid 4 grams t.i.d., niacinamide 500 mg t.i.d., B-complex 50s od, selenium 200 mcg t.i.d., beta carotene 25,000 iu per day, zinc citrate 50 mg od, cod liver oil 2 capsules per day, evening primrose oil 2 capsules per day, germanium 1 tablet b.i.d., vitamin E 800 iu per day.

She was seen again in June 1990. She was on ascorbic acid 16 grams per day plus the rest of the program. She had no pain, her weight was steady, and she was not depressed. Beta carotene was increased to 75,000 iu t.i.d.. In August 1990 she reported she was following the entire program, the lump was getting smaller, and she felt well, although she was still concerned over her blindness. In November 1990 she reported she planned to get chelation therapy and that the lump was smaller. She telephoned in April 1991 to discuss a social problem she was having, and called my secretary in December 1991 to report she was doing well; she was concerned, however, that her family physician, who herself had been receiving standard therapy for breast cancer for the past year, was not doing well at all and had given up her practice.

She called in early February 1992 to report she was doing well. She had sold her house and was moving to an apartment in a nearby community. On 30 November 1992 she was free of cancer but was having other physical problems which had put her into hospital several times over the summer. On 4 August 1993 she was free of cancer. In July 1996 she was well.

(3) Case #175

Born in 1948, she was first seen in March 1990. This patient had a lumpectomy, right side. She had detected a lump some time before that, noticeable just before her periods, and her breasts were tender. Mammogram suggested a cyst but biopsy was positive for cancer. Further exploration was suggested and radiation was considered. She had been under a lot of stress over the past year. I started her on the following program: ascorbic acid 4 t.i.d., chromium 500 mcg per day, niacinamide 500 mg t.i.d., B-complex 50s od, pyridoxine 100 mg od, zinc citrate 50 mg b.i.d., selenium 200 mcg t.i.d., magnesium oxide 420 mg od, calcium 500 mg per day, evening primrose oil 3 capsules per day, beta carotene 25,000 iu per day, cod liver oil 3 capsules per day, vitamin E 800 iu per day, folic acid 5 mg b.i.d.

She reported on 30 May 1990 that she had had a lumpectomy April 12th and one node was positive. She had just started chemotherapy and would be receiving it every three weeks. She would also receive radiation between chemotherapy sessions. She felt great and had come through the operation easily. At that time her beta carotene was increased to 25,000 iu t.i.d. and she was on sodium ascorbate 12 to 15 g per day.

On 13 February 1992 she was normal, on the entire program, was cheerful, and there had been no recurrences. On 17 November 1992 she was well and cheerful and remained well in February 1996.

(4) Case #188

Born in 1945, she was first seen in May 1989. Following her annual medical checkup when she had a mammogram, a tumor of the left breast was discovered. It was less than 2 cm in diameter, and she received a lumpectomy with axillary dissection in early March 1989. There were no positive nodes (stage 1). She had never been ill and was quite surprised when this happened. Her surgeon had recommended radiation after surgery, but no chemotherapy was suggested. Because she was tense after her biopsy, she was given valium, to which she had a very severe reaction lasting 7 days, including phlebitis, joint pains, etc. She had to receive two different types of antibiotics in order to deal with this reaction because it was thought she might have some kind of hidden infection.

She had heard about the use of nutrition and supplements to enhance the immune system, and wanted to do what she could to help herself. I suggested she start on the following program: ascorbic acid 4 grams t.i.d., niacinamide 500 mg t.i.d., B-complex 50s od, vitamin A 20,000 iu per day, beta carotene 20,000 iu per day, zinc citrate 50 mg per day, magnesium oxide 420 mg od, selenium 200 mcg b.i.d., vitamin E 400 iu b.i.d. She was to continue eltroxin 125 mcg per day.

On 21 June 1989 she reported she had more energy, was no longer exhausted, and could tolerate the whole program. She had some pain in the left axilla. It was decided she did not require radiation. Kelp 1 g b.i.d. was added to her program. On 18 February 1992 she reported she was well and was following the whole program. She was cheerful and had in the meantime remarried. In May 1996 she was well.

(5) Case #201

Born in 1946, she was first seen in May 1990. In 1986 this patient developed a lump in her left breast which was biopsied and found to be benign in February 1987. However, a second lump formed beneath the scar tissue, and in July 1989 was found malignant. She was given a lumpectomy, followed in September 1989 by mastectomy. Four nodes were positive of 17 examined. In October 1989 she started chemotherapy every three weeks. In January 1990 she had 16 radiation sessions and felt very sick thereafter, having her last treatment January 25. After that she improved but she still lacked energy.

She was started on the following program: ascorbic acid 4 grams t.i.d., niacinamide 500 mg t.i.d., B-complex 50s od, vitamin E 400 iu b.i.d., beta carotene 25,000 iu t.i.d., cod liver oil 6 capsules per day, selenium 200 mcg t.i.d., zinc citrate 50 mg od, cal/mag 2 tablets b.i.d., folic acid 5 mg od, Slow-K 600 mg b.i.d. Late in November 1990 she reported she was doing well, was still following her diet, but had reduced her vitamin intake. She felt well, was working full time, keeping very busy, and she was optimistic. She contacted me again in December 1991 to report she was very well and free of cancer. She remained on her vitamin program. On 31 March 1993 she wrote that there had been an increase in tumor markers and that she had been started on tamoxifen. In May 1994 she wrote that she was well and working. Her tumor blood marker was slightly elevated. In May 1996 she was well.

(6) Case #208
Born in 1936, she was first seen in December 1988. In March 1988 a lump was detected in her right breast which was positive on biopsy; there also had been some spread to the glands on that side. She refused surgery, putting herself, instead, on a very good program including herbs. Later she went to the Hoxey Clinic in Mexico for a vaccine treatment, which did not help, and eventually went to the Gerson Clinic in Mexico for three weeks of treatment. The cancer continued to grow and eventually her arm was three times its normal size, with the breast very large and the tumor very prominent. She then consulted a physician who started her on IV vitamin C 50 grams per day, gradually increasing it to 75 grams per day. Apparently, the swelling in her arm and breast disappeared soon after starting the injections, and the tumor began to recede very quickly. She also had had one chemotherapy treatment about that time. Bone scan was negative. She was healing quite well and both she and her husband were quite optimistic.

She was on a daily regimen of vitamin E 1,500 iu, vitamin A 4,000 iu, vitamin D 400 iu, B-complex 25s, kelp 4 tablets, and selenium 200 mcg. She was not able to take more than 9 grams per day of vitamin C orally because of diarrhea, and was also taking B-12 injections 1 mg every three weeks. I modified her program as follows: to continue her IV ascorbate, add calcium ascorbate 4 grams t.i.d. if possible, niacinamide 500 mg t.i.d., beta carotene 20,000 iu per day, selenium 200 mcg t.i.d., magnesium oxide 420 mg per day.

In July 1989 she reported she had had her last chemotherapy in June, and that she had not been too sick on treatment days. She was on intravenous ascorbate 25 grams once per week as well as 12-16 grams per day orally. She had had one radiation treatment, her hair was coming back, the hard tissue she had in her axilla was clearing, and her mood was good. Her program was modified to niacin 50 mg t.i.d., vitamin E 800 iu per day, selenium 200 mcg b.i.d., beta carotene 50,000 iu per day, vitamin C 20 grams per day, evening primrose oil 2 capsules per day, and lecithin 1.2 g per day. Early in 1991 she started ozone therapy. When I spoke with her on 20 February 1992, she was still well with no sign of any recurrence. On 12 January 1994 she was still well and still receiving ozone treatments. A recent check up showed no evidence for any cancer. In July 1996 she was well.

(7) Case #209

Born in 1936, she was first seen in March 1989. The previous year, about one month after detecting a lump in her right breast, she received a radical mastectomy. No nodes were involved, but there had been some spread to the vascular system, and she was not sure if it had been adherent to the skin. After that she received six months of chemotherapy, one treatment every three weeks, followed by 22 radiation treatments, the last in May 1988. She had been following a vitamin program of her own for some time to try to prevent a recurrence.

She had gone through a difficult period with digestive problems about five years before, to the point she consulted the Mayo Clinic. She was treated by food avoidance to try to pinpoint her food allergies and this was not a major problem when I saw her. She did have hot flashes since her radiation and complained that her joints had been aching.

I started her on the following program: ascorbic acid 4 g t.i.d., niacinamide 500 mg t.i.d., B-complex 50s od, vitamin E 800 iu per day, pyridoxine 100 mg per day, vitamin A 10,000 iu per day, selenium 200 mcg t.i.d., beta carotene 20,000 iu per day, cal/mag (500 mg calcium/250 mg magnesium) per day.

On 20 February 1992, she reported she was well, with no sign of any recurrence. Her mood was good. In July 1996 she was well.

(8) Case #236

Born in 1941, she was first seen in January 1989. In October 1987 this patient developed a lump in her left breast, which examination and mammogram indicated was cystic. She had had problems with the breast for the previous 12 years. In 1988, because the cyst persisted, it was aspirated and found negative, but later biopsy indicated she was positive for cancer. She received a lumpectomy on 1 December 1988; all glands were negative. It was recommended that she have chemotherapy because of estrogen sensitivity, but she was loath to do because of possible side effects, especially on her eyes, and she had not yet made a decision.

I suggested she start on the following: calcium ascorbate 2 grams t.i.d., ascorbic acid 2 t.i.d., vitamin E 400 iu per day, B-complex 50s od, niacinamide 500 mg t.i.d., beta carotene 20,000 iu, calcium 1000 mg per day, magnesium 500 mg per day, and zinc citrate 50 mg od. In March 1989 she was on the whole program and was receiving chemotherapy every four weeks and would receive a total of 9. Her oncologist told her he was pleased she was on a vitamin program. On 23 March 1992, the family doctor who had referred her to me indicated she was well and had moved to Vancouver. In January 1996 she was well.

(9) Case #250

Born in 1955, she was first seen in July 1989. In December 1988 she became aware of soreness of the right nipple. She became pregnant, but on 4 May 1989, the breast became red, hard and swollen, with a large lump. She was examined by ultrasound and placed on antibiotics for 30 days altogether, first on ampicillin, then on cloxicillin, without any improvement. At this time also her skin became kind of puckered. Biopsy revealed an adenocarcinoma; one lymph gland was involved. The tumor was mobile without any adhesion to skin or underlying tissues.

Shortly after that she received a therapeutic abortion, having been advised that carrying the fetus to term might cost her her life. The tumor appeared to be growing very quickly. She had two young children at home. She was then started on chemotherapy, having received 3 or 4 treatments by the time I saw her. She was on a variable schedule, and after the first set of chemotherapy it was planned to give her four weeks of radiation therapy, followed by another 12 weeks of chemotherapy. She had few ill effects from the chemotherapy.

I started her on the following program: ascorbic acid 2 g t.i.d., calcium ascorbate 2 g t.i.d., niacinamide 500 mg t.i.d., B-complex 50s mg od, folic acid 5 mg b.i.d., beta carotene 20,000 iu per day, selenium 200 mcg b.i.d., vitamin E 400 iu b.i.d., zinc citrate 50 mg od, kelp 3 tablets per day, magnesium oxide 420 mg per day, cal/mag 2 per day, and coenzyme Q_{10} 30 mg t.i.d.

On 31 August 1989, she reported she was able to follow the whole program. She was receiving radiation. She felt fine and her mood was good. I heard from her again in December 1990, and she was still doing well with no recurrences. On 1 November 1992 she was normal and planned on becoming pregnant again. In July 13, 1993 the cancer recurred with lesions in both lungs, mostly at the base. She was given taxol and cisplatin. On 16

December 1993 she had nearly completed the treatment. She felt much better and was optimistic. I then advised her to increase her Q_{10} to 320 mg daily. She was still on the vitamin program.

On 4 March 1996 she told me several metastases had been found in her brain, for which she had just completed radiation treatment. Her mood was good. I suggested she add bovine cartilage 9 g daily to her program, melatonin 21 mg od, flax seed oil , 2 tablespoonfuls. In September 1996 she was alive.

(10) Case #278

Born in 1943, she was first seen in July 1988. Around July 1985 she detected a lump in her breast. In November 1985 she had a modified radical mastectomy. Three nodes out of 12 were positive. Following that she was given 6 chemotherapy sessions over a 9 month period and 16 radiation treatments over a period of 3 weeks. She had a minor radiation burn on her skin. She consulted me in order to find out how she could decrease the chance for a recurrence.

I advised her to take ascorbic acid 6 g, niacin 1.5 g, B-complex 50s, folic acid 5 mg b.i.d., zinc gluconate 50 mg, vitamin E 800 iu, beta carotene 20,000 iu, selenium 200 mcg t.i.d., and thyroid 60 mg, all daily. On 4 July 1994 she was well and was still following this program. In July 1996 she was well.

– Abram Hoffer

Prostate Cancer

Summary

The prostate is the gland surrounding the urethra at the base of the bladder in males that secretes an alkaline fluid that makes up part of the semen and enhances the motility and fertility of sperm. Enlargement of the prostate is a common accompaniment of the aging process, indicated by obstruction to the voiding of urine, increased frequency of urination, and a feeling of incomplete emptying of the bladder. Most of these prostatic problems are benign, but a fraction are malignant, and this fraction increases with advancing years. Digital rectal examination can usually distinguish malignant from benign enlargement, and biochemical tests can be used to confirm the diagnosis.

The usual treatment of benign enlargement is surgery and that of malignant enlargement is the administration of hormones. Prostatic cancer metastasizes to the bones, each metastasis causing local pain. When hormonal treatment fails, radiotherapy and chemotherapy may produce favorable response. There is evidence for the effectiveness of megavitamin and other orthomolecular treatments.

– Linus Pauling

In Canada, prostate cancer constitutes 24 percent of the total cases of all cancers.

By the end of 1995 I had seen 48 patients with prostate cancer. The survival data is shown in Table 21. By the end of 1990, 18 patients were seen and had they all survived they would have reached the five year cure. Only 11 or 61 percent did. But the patients seen by the end of 1991 only had a 4 year follow-up period. Out of this group, 15 or 60 percent were alive. Only 3 patients were not on the nutrition regimen. One lived 5 years and the other 2 died the first year.

– Abram Hoffer

Survival Rates

In a review of research on prostate cancer by W.J. Catalona, it was reported that stage T1 and T2 patients, after treatment, had the same survival expectancy as the general population. Stage 3 cases have a survival expectancy which is 25 to 50 percent lower than the rate in the general population. Stage 4 cases with node involvement and metastases have a very poor prognosis, probably lower than 25 percent. The three prostate patients in this small series had a survival rate much lower than the vitamin treated group and probably provides a crude estimate of the kind of patients that were referred to me.

– Abram Hoffer

Lymphomas

Summary

The lymphatic system is comprised of the body-wide system of lymphatic vessels, which drain into many lymph nodes, and transporting lymph, which is a transparent slightly yellowish coagulable fluid containing white blood cells (lymphocytes) in a fluid resembling blood plasma. The main source of the lymphocytes is the spleen. This whole system is actively engaged in protection against cancer, and it is interesting that metastases to the spleen rarely occur. Some constituent cells of the lymphatic system, which also includes the tonsils and the thymus gland, may themselves become malignant, producing the kinds of cancer called the lymphomas. There are many kinds of lymphomas, including lymphosarcoma, reticulum-cell sarcoma, and Hodgkins disease. They are the fifth most deadly kind of cancer, causing about 25,000 deaths per year (not including lymphatic leukemia) in the United States.

TABLE 21

The Survival By Years of All Prostate Cancer Patients on The Vitamin Regimen and on Standard Treatment Only Seen Between 1978 and the end of 1993.

On Orthomolecular Plus Standard Treatment					Standard Only		
Year Seen	Years could have lived	Number at risk	Alive at end of year	Percent alive	N	Alive	%
1994	1	41	35	85	There were three controls. Two died the first year and one in the seventh year.		
1993	2	35	27	77			
1992	3	28	19	68			
1991	4	25	15	60			
1990	5	18	11	61			
1989	6	14	9	64			
1988	7	11	2	18			
1987	8	8	2	25			
1986	9	4	1	25			
1985	10	0					

There is some indication of a viral origin of lymphomas and leukemia, in that clusters of cases seem to occur in precise geographical regions, down to certain streets in certain towns, and similar diseases in animals are caused by viruses. People exposed to high-energy radiation have a greatly increased incidence of lymphomas and leukemia.

Until a couple of decades ago these malignancies were uniformly fatal. Today, thanks to the combined use of radiotherapy and chemotherapy, a significant proportion of patients with these diseases can be cured. Moreover, there is evidence that orthomolecular methods are also valuable with the lymphomas and leukemias.

– Linus Pauling

Survival Rates

Male patients had an edge in survival compared to females, as shown in Table 23. From 15 male patients, there was 1 death the first year, 1 in the second year, 1 in the third year, and 1 in the fifth year. Eleven are alive today. From 7 female patients, there were 2 deaths the first year, 4 the second year, and 1 in the third year.

Case Histories

Cases Alive Ten or More Years

(1) Case #11

Born in 1959, he was first seen in March 1984. On 24 December 1982 he complained of acute left upper quadrant pain. His white blood count was 15,000 and he had some fever. He recovered in a few days. On 11 February 1983 he was found to have a huge abdominal mass on the left side. After a few days he left hospital before the investigation was completed but came back a few days later. A few days later he was started on chemotherapy, and by 3 March 1983 the mass was smaller and softer. But his oncologist recorded that "he presents with an incurable condition which undoubtedly in the near future will take him away." He was then diagnosed as having paranoid schizophrenia with retroperitoneal lymphoma.

TABLE 22

Prostate Cancer Survivors

Seen by year end	Number Seen	Years following first visit. Alive — Number Alive					Percent
		1	2	3	4	5	
1990	18					11	61
1991	25				15		60
1992	28			19			68
1993	35		27				77
1994	41	35					85

TABLE 23

The Survival By Years of Lymphoma Patients on The Vitamin Regimen and on Standard Treatment Only, Seen Between 1978 and the end of 1993

On Orthomolecular Plus Standard Treatment					Standard Only
Year Seen	Years could have lived	Number at risk	Alive at end of year	Percent alive	
1994	1	22	19	86	
1993	2	19	11	58	
1992	3	16	8	50	
1991	4	16	8	50	
1990	5	10	6	60	One control died in the first year, the other in the second year.
1989	6	7	4	57	
1988	7	6	4	67	
1987	8	3	3	100	
1986	9	3	3	100	
1985	10	3	3	100	

On 27 March 1984 I examined him. He was very anxious and worried about his lymphoma. He was then not showing any schizophrenic symptoms and signs. I started him on ascorbic acid 12 g, niacin 1.5 g, B-complex 75s, twice daily, and selenium 150 mcg, all daily. On 4 February 1985 he was admitted to the psychiatric ward. This time he complained of visual illusions, he had a few paranoid delusions, and was very depressed. He was admitted again in March 1985, and by then I had rediagnosed him with schizophrenia, paranoid. He was started on a parenteral slow release tranquilizer because he was not very good at following his medication regimen. He was admitted for the last time July 1991 for two days following several experiences with LSD. He had had many admissions over the previous 6 years. For his schizophrenia and to prevent a recurrence of the lymphoma, he took niacin between 3 and 12 g daily, ascorbic acid between 3 and 20 g daily, and any medication he needed using antidepressants or tranquilizers.

At the end of 1993 he was free of his lymphoma but his mental condition was unknown. When last seen he was on niacin 6 g and ascorbic acid 20 g, daily. He was alive 30 June 1996, but I have not seen him for several years.

(2) Case # 66

Born in 1970, he was first seen in February 1984. He became sick in 1979, diagnosed with Crohn's disease. He was given prednisone and stopped growing. His bowel ruptured and required surgery. Two years later he developed Hodgkins lymphoma with the tumors in his abdomen. He was given a 10 percent chance of survival. He received chemotherapy with severe side effects, losing all his hair. He would have had surgery but was too weak. His mother then started him a on a comprehensive dietary mineral vitamin program including laetrile.

I saw him 20 February 1984 and advised him to remain on his program but to include ascorbic acid 3 g, vitamin E 200 iu, selenium 200 mcg, and vitamin A 50,000 iu, all daily. When last contact was made, he had graduated from university and had remained well. He was not following the vitamin program regularly. He continued to improve and was well at 10 years after I first saw him. I took him off the follow-up list. However, on 23 November 1996 I ran into his parents in downtown Victoria. They told me that he is still well and they were very grateful for this.

(3) Case #74

Born in 1947, he was first seen in January 1982. He was severely depressed. I started him on an antidepressant and on ascorbic acid 3 g and niacin 3 g daily. On 2 December 1982 he was operated for a mass on his back which was found to be benign; however, he did not feel good and the surgical area would not heal. After further surgery his wound began to heal. In May 1983 he began to suffer severe abdominal pain and was constipated. In June 1983 biopsy of his spleen showed a lymphoma, a small cell diffuse lyphocytic lymphoma described as controllable, not curable. He was given cobalt radiotherapy. I increased his ascorbic acid to 12 g, adding selenium 400 mcg, vitamin E 400 iu, and magnesium oxide 840 mg.

In July 1983 he started to receive chemotherapy – adriamyacin, cyclophosphamide, vincristine, and prednisone – receiving six cycles. In February 1984 he was started on radiotherapy, 15 sessions over three weeks. On his own he increased his selenium to 2,000 mcg daily. There were no side effects, but I asked him to decrease it to 1,000 mcg. On 16 March 1984 he had a diffuse mass posteriorly on the left side of his chest wall. He was given more radiation therapy in 15 sessions. On May 22 the mass was gone, but on June 11 it had recurred as a paraspinal mass of the lower left thoracic spine, separate from the previous mass. He was given more chemotherapy and radiotherapy, completed in May 29. By then he had a left sided effusion lymphoma infiltrate. On 25 June 1984 more nodes were developing. The oncologist noted that he "clearly has a progressive disease not being controlled by chlorambucil and prednisone." On 5 July 1984 he received more chemotherapy with a dramatic resolution of the glands. In August 1984, still on chemotherapy, his oncologist recorded that "I can definitely state that this man has persistent incurable malignant disease."

By 24 September 1984 he was free of symptoms and refused to accept any more chemotherapy. On 23 January 1985 a CT scan showed a large right pelvic mass and a second smaller one near the duodenal loop. He was given more radiotherapy to the mass. On 19 April 19 1985 a 2 cm diameter mass appeared in his right leg. This was his eighth recurrence of cancer.

By March 1986 he had recovered. In April 1988 he was well. His oncologist knew he was taking vitamins and was unhappy about this. He recorded 3 August 1983, "I can no longer feel any intra-abdominal mass. Unfortunately, he started on large doses of vitamin C and B vitamins prior to therapy and he is convinced that these are responsible for his good response rather than the chemotherapy." On 31 December 1994 he was well and on the regimen. He is a poet and wrote a poem to celebrate his recovery after he had been given three months of life at the most after he was diagnosed. In September 1966 he was well. This patient is normal, has established a good relationship with a woman he met in Victoria, has a job, and is active in community affairs. During his last visit to me several months ago, I asked him how much vitamin C he had been able to take. He replied that he had been on 40 g daily. He said that he had severe diarrhea and had to sit on the toilet most of the day reading, but that considering the alternative he did not mind. In fact, vitamin C does not produce the usual type of diarrhea common to severe abdominal infections. It simply makes the stools very watery due to retention of water. It is more like a continuous excretion of watery stools but will not cause dehydration if the fluid intake is maintained.

Hodgkins Disease

Eight patients were treated. One died after five years. One did not reach five years. Her history is given below. The rest are still alive, ranging from 2 to 6 years.

(1) Case # 355
Born in 1950, she was first seen in December 1991. One year before I saw her she developed night sweats. Later she was found to have a mass in her chest and one in her neck. She was given chemotherapy for six months in 21 day cycles. Following that she had one month of radiation. She was very sick during the chemotherapy, was very tired, and developed sores in her mouth. When I saw her, she was much better. On prednisone she had gained much weight. In addition, she was depressed. I advised her to take ascorbic acid 12 g, niacinamide 1.5 g, B-complex 50, selenium 600 mcg, beta carotene 25,000 iu, zinc citrate 50 mg, all daily.

On 11 August 1994 she was normal, but on 16 February 1996 she died suddenly. However, she did not die directly because of her cancer: the cause of death was status post chemotherapy and mediastianal radiation for nodular sclerosing Hodgkins disease given in 1991. Her heart showed

Adriamycin-induced cardiotoxicity, with a resulting dilated cardiomyopathy and mural thrombus formation within the right atrium and right ventricle. Perhaps if she had not had this severe toxic reaction to the chemotherapy, she would still be alive today.

– Abram Hoffer

Bladder and Kidney Cancer

Summary

Cancer of the bladder causes about 12,000 deaths per year in the United States, 8,000 of them in males. It ranges from almost innocuous benign warty growths to solid ulcerated deeply invasive tumors. During an illness with bladder cancer, which may last for many years, there is a relentless increase in the degree of malignancy. The disease is multifocal: the whole bladder lining is pre-malignant, so that even if one lesion is successfully treated, others are likely to appear. The disease is usually recognized by the observation of blood in the urine.

The association of bladder cancer with certain industrial chemicals is well established. There is also an increased incidence with heavy tobacco smoking and coffee drinking, and in certain persons with an inborn error in the metabolism of the amino acid tryptophan. All of these circumstances result in the excretion of chemical carcinogens in the urine. For some of these carcinogens, it has been shown that vitamin C has a significant protective effect; accordingly, the orthomolecular regimen, as an adjunct to appropriate conventional therapy, will help significantly in controlling the disease. The conventional therapy is surgery and sometimes the use of high-energy radiation.

Cancer of the kidney is rather rare, causing only about 8,000 deaths per year in the United States. The common form of kidney cancer is usually recognized from the presence of blood in the urine, often with a dull dragging discomfort in the affected loin, and is verified by radiography. Treatment is by surgical removal of the whole tumor-bearing kidney.

As the untreated or unsuspected disease progresses, however, metastases form in the bones and the lung. Radiotherapy and chemotherapy have been found to have little value, but orthomolecular treatment may succeed in controlling the cancer.

– Linus Pauling

Case Histories

There were 7 cases of bladder cancer in this series of cases. Two died the first year, one from a coronary occlusion. One died in the second, one in the third and one in the sixth year. Two are alive.

There were 13 cases of kidney cancer. All of the 3 controls died in the first year. From the 10 that were on the regimen, 7 were alive one year, 5 were alive 2 years, one lived 4 years and one 8 years. Five are still living, range 2 to 8 years. For both bladder and kidney cancers, the cases living more than 4 years are recorded here.

Bladder

(1) Case # 24

Born in 1921, she was first seen in March 1983. After she had been bleeding from her bladder for 4 months, a carcinoma was diagnosed. The tumor had penetrated the bladder wall. She was given 15 radiation treatments, the last in March 1983. I started her on ascorbic acid 5 g t.i.d., niacin 500 mg t.i.d., pyridoxine 200 mg od, zinc sulfate 220 mg od, selenium 300 mcg b.i.d., and magnesium oxide 410 mg b.i.d. One month after she had increased the ascorbic acid to 16 g daily. In September 1986 the tumor recurred after she had decreased her ascorbic acid intake to 1 g per day several months before. She developed pain in her left hip in December 1987 and was considered terminal. On 30 March 1988 she increased her ascorbic acid to 12 g od. She died in August 1988.

Kidney

(1) Case #126

Born in 1945, she was first seen in October 1987. When I first saw her, she told me that metastases from her kidney had invaded her femur, causing a lot of pain. She received 10 radiation treatments and the pain was relieved.

I started her on ascorbic acid 4 g t.i.d., niacin 500 mg t.i.d., selenium 200 mcg b.i.d., magnesium oxide 420 mg od, zinc gluconate 50 mg od, beta carotene 50,000 id od, A B complex 50s preparation od, and vitamin E 800 iu od. In November 1986 her right leg was amputated. The following April she was getting on well and was following the regimen. She was still well in September 1996.

(2) Case #312

Born in 1948, she was first seen in August 1991. In June 1991 she developed persistent pain so severe she went to the emergency room of the hospital. On June 14 a mass was removed from her kidney. It had not spread and she was given a good prognosis. She was, however, very worried about a relapse and came to talk about the use of vitamins. I advised her to take vitamin C 8 g, niacinamide 1 g, B complex (50), selenium 400 mcg, and beta carotene 50,000 iu. One year later she was normal. No recurrence was found at her annual check up. She was well September 1996.

(3) Case #443

Born in 1988, he was first seen in June 1992. In February 1991 his father noted a mass on his right side. Wilms tumor was diagnosed and the right kidney mass was removed plus about 5 inches of intestine. He also had 5 spots in his lungs and was started on chemotherapy, one session per week for twelve weeks. In May 1991 two masses were removed from his lungs and he was then given radiation for two more still present. He was very small, weighing 22 pounds, his sense of taste was poor, and he had no appetite. His parents had to force him to eat. He had white areas in his finger nails, indicating a serious zinc deficiency. I advised his parents to start him on ascorbic acid. He could not swallow anything and so had to be given chewable vitamin C. They were able to give him 500 mg daily. He was also given liquid zinc sulfate 30 mg daily. On 11 January 1993 he was normal. His mother told me he had had a recent cancer check up six months following his last chemotherapy and there was no evidence of any recurrence. She added that his appetite became normal only after he started taking the zinc solution.

On 14 February 1994 a CT scan showed another tumor in the left lung. On 6 July 1994 the tumor had not grown any more and appeared a little smaller on examination. He was taking 8 g of vitamin C plus the other vitamins. I added pycnogenol 40 mg o.d. to his program. He felt well and appeared normal. In June 1996 he was normal. He was clear of cancer.

– Abram Hoffer

Leukemias

Summary

Leukemia is a kind of malignancy characterized by the appearance of enormous numbers of white cells in the circulating blood. There are two main forms of leukemia which are classified according to the primary cell type, lymphatic leukemia and myeloid leukemia. Lymphatic leukemia arises from a primary malignancy of the lymphatic system and the circulating blood contains an immense number of lymphocytes, whereas myeloid leukemia arises from the leukocyte-forming cells of the bone marrow and the blood contains other kinds of white cells called granulocytes. Each category is further divided into acute and chronic, depending on the degree of malignancy. The acute leukemias often occur in children.

The symptoms of leukemia are increasing lassitude, anemia, ease of bruising, susceptibility to infections, loss of weight, night sweats, enlargement of the spleen and sometimes the liver, and, for lymphatic leukemia, swelling of the lymph nodes. Differential diagnosis is made by a blood-cell count. As with the lymphomas, leukemia can now often be cured by radiotherapy and chemotherapy, but such successful treatment requires special expertise and often special hospital facilities.

The symptoms of acute leukemia are identical to the symptoms of scurvy. It is well established that the circulating white cells in leukemia are abnormally low in their content of vitamin C. This suggests that correction of this deficit might be beneficial to the leukemia patients, and there is evidence of the value of orthomolecular treatment.

– Linus Pauling

Case Histories

Out of 16 patients in the study with leukemia, 10 were alive one year, 9 were alive 2 years, 5 were alive 3 years, 4 were alive 4 years, 3 were alive 5 years, and 6 are still living.

(1) Case #94

Born in 1920, she was first seen in August 1983. In 1958 this patient was treated for goiter with radioactive iodine, after which she needed thyroid hormone and calcium to prevent severe muscle cramps. In March 1983 chronic leukemia was found. When I saw her, she also complained that she had severe pain in her hands and feet, swollen fingers, a dry scaly skin, and angina not related to effort. I advised her to add ascorbic acid 1 g t.i.d., niacin 1 g t.i.d., pyridoxine 250 mg od, zinc gluconate 100 mg od, and flax seed oil 1 tablespoonful od. Two months after her blood picture was much better and she felt better. The pain had diminished. After another month her platelet count increased to about 250,000, her white blood cells count decreased from 11,200 to 9,100, and her hemoglobin increased from 13.4 to 14.0 G. A CT scan showed that liver and spleen were enlarged. By April 1988 she was much better. Her liver and spleen were normal as was her blood count but her feet still hurt. She felt good and was cheerful. She died in December 1989, age 69.

(2) Case #104

Born in 1924, he was first seen in November 1987. Following mild fatigue present for 1.5 years, hairy leukemia was diagnosed in February 1987. After I saw him, he started on ascorbic acid 4 g t.i.d., niacin 0.5 g t.i.d., folic acid 5 mg od, selenium 200 mcg t.i.d., beta carotene 20,000 i.u. od, zinc citrate 100 mg od, a vitamin B-complex 50s preparation od, magnesium oxide 420 mg od, and cod liver oil capsules t.i.d. He started chemotherapy in 1988, completing the series in July. By April 1989 he was well and taking only ascorbic acid 8 g daily. When he was first seen in November, hemoglobin was 11.6, then by April hemoglobin was 12.2, wbc was 2,900, platelets were 86,000, and there were 15 percent circulating hairy cells. By February 1989 his hemoglobin was 14.2, his wbc 6,000, and there were no hairy leukocytes. He was still well in October 1996.

(3) Case #307

Born in 1916, he was first seen in June 1991. He had a triple coronary bypass 12 years earlier and later had a pacemaker inserted. In August 1990 chronic leukemia was diagnosed. He started himself on a mixture of vitamins and minerals. His wife died the previous November from cancer of the breast.

In February 1991 he suffered a heart attack and was placed upon medication. When I saw him, I advised him to follow the program he was on, but to include vitamin C 12 g, niacin 1.5 g, pyridoxine 250 mg, vitamin E 800 iu, selenium 600 mcg, zinc citrate 50 mg, and beta carotene 25,000 iu, all daily. On May 20 1992 I added l-lysine 2 g daily. In June 1992 his white cell count was stable, around 10 g/L. On 28 January 1993 his blood platelets were low, but the rest of the count was normal. His mood was good. I added folic acid 10 mg and vitamin B-12 1 mg daily to his program. He was still well in July 1996.

(3) Case #311
Born in 1912, she was first seen in July 1986. This patient came to see me because of her severe arthritis present for 13 years. She had started herself on a multivitamin program and felt better but wanted advice on how to improve this. She then told me she had chronic lymphatic leukemia, her wbc being 16.7 in July 1984 and remaining at that level since. She had her spleen, gall bladder, and appendix removed. I added niacinamide 1.5 g daily for her arthritis. She was already taking vitamin C 6 g , selenium 200 mcg, and other nutrients. In February 1987 I increased her niacin to 4 g daily. By March 1988, she was free of pain. In May 1987 she had surgery to remove a small bowel blockage and was given a temporary colostomy. I saw her in September 1989 and she was getting on very well. When seen last by her general practitioner at the end of January 1992, her mood was good, but she was still having some difficulty with her arthritis. She was still on her vitamin program. She was still well in July 1996.

– Abram Hoffer

Pancreas Cancer

Summary

Pancreatic cancer is rather common, causing about 25,000 deaths per year in the United States. It occurs about twice as often in cigarette smokers as in non-smokers. There are two kinds of cancer of the pancreas, one located at the head of the pancreas (the most common kind), the other in the body of the pancreas. The bile duct, which conveys a waste product from the liver to the intestines, passes through the head of the pancreas, and a pancreatic cancer at that site blocks the flow of the bile, causing pain, jaundice (yellow color to the skin and eyes), intense itch, the passage of pale yellow stools and dark urine. Surgical removal of the pancreas is risky and is rarely carried out, but a simple by-pass operation can reconnect the bile duct to the intestines, causing the jaundice to clear, and the patient may then enjoy reasonably good health for months and even years.

Cancer of the body of the pancreas is hard to diagnose because the symptoms are vague – diminishing appetite, loss of weight, upper abdominal discomfort, and backache. There is no known effective conventional therapy for this form of cancer, but orthomolecular treatment has been found to be effective in a number of patients.

– Linus Pauling

Case Histories

The series contained 10 patients with cancer of the pancreas. Six died the first year, 1 died in the second year, and 2 were still alive at 18 and 9 years. Nine were in the control group. They all died within 5 months, averaging 2 months after they first saw me. Dr Pauling's analysis of the first 4 cases led to the conclusion that the excellent responders would survive between 13 and 30 times as long as the control group. So far out of 10 patients, the present survival is 48 months, or 24 times the survival of the control group.

Cases Living More Than Two Years

(1) Case #58

Born in 1922, she was first seen in November 1986. In 1984 she began to suffer repeated episodes of weakness. One year later her glands became swollen and her stools became very pale. In October 1986 she was given a bypass after becoming severely jaundiced. I improved her diet and started her on ascorbic acid 4 g t.i.d., niacinamide 500 mg t.i.d., beta carotene 10,000 iu b.i.d., vitamin A 25,000 iu od, zinc sulfate 220 mg od, and selenium 200 mcg t.i.d. One month later she had been able to increase her ascorbic acid level to 22 g od. In October 1996 she was still well 10 years later.

(2) Case #84

Born in 1919, she was first seen in July 1978. In May 1978 she developed obstructive jaundice. At laparotomy a 6 cm diameter hard mass was found in the head of the pancreas which totally obstructed her common bile duct. The diagnosis was so certain it was decided not to do a biopsy in order not to increase the chance of metastases. A cholecysto-jejunostomy was performed. After the operation she was informed her prognosis was very poor and that she should get her affairs in order. She had been concerned about cancer for three years following the death of her sister.

She was determined that she would not die. She had read Norman Cousins's book, Anatomy of an Illness, where he described his recovery using megadoses of ascorbic acid (intravenously at first, later orally) and laughter induced by watching funny movies. She began to take 12 to 16 g daily plus small amounts of B vitamins. On 21 July 1978 I advised her to increase her ascorbic acid to bowel tolerance levels and to add niacinamide 1.5 g, zinc sulfate 220 mg, and proteolytic enzymes with each meal. She went up to 40 g but one month later was taking only 35 g daily. On 21 February 1979 she told me that a recent CT scan had shown no mass was present. The radiologist could not believe this and repeated the scan with the same results. A few months later another scan showed that her common bile duct was functioning well. She now has two. She remained on the whole program for five years, then decreased the amount of ascorbic acid she was taking. In June 1996 she was well.

This patient told her friends and her co-workers about her recovery. Soon some of them were referred to me and gradually the number of referrals increased. I credit this patient with having brought me into this new field which might be termed orthomolecular oncology.

– Abram Hoffer

Cervix, Uterus, and Ovary Cancer

Summary

Cancer of the uterine cervix, the neck of the uterus, causes about 4,000 deaths per year. It can be detected, even in the premalignant stage, by examination of the Pap smear, with gynecological examination if there is suspicion of a positive reading. Surgery and radiotherapy are effective, except when the malignancy has infiltrated the adjacent tissues.

Cancer of the body of the uterus causes about 4,000 deaths per year. It occurs most frequently around the menopausal age. It is recognized by menstrual irregularity, post-menopausal bleeding, and abnormally heavy menstrual periods. Unless the disease has already spread beyond the limit of surgery, the treatment is hysterectomy, resulting in a high rate of cure. Cancer of the ovary causes about 12,000 deaths per year in the United States. There are many types of ovarian cancer, some much more malignant than others. The initial treatment is surgical removal of the tumor, both ovaries, and the uterus. Metastases occur to the liver and throughout the abdominal cavity, producing a massive accumulation of fluid (ascites). Some ovarian cancers show good response to radiotherapy or chemotherapy, and there is good evidence for the value of orthomolecular treatment.

– Linus Pauling

Case Histories

Patients with Cancer of the Uterus Surviving 8 or More Years

(1) Case #19

Born in 1943, she was first seen in February 1983. In 1972 she had an hysterectomy and oophorectomy for cancer of the uterus, followed by radiation. In 1981 carcinoma in situ on the labia was treated surgically. After I saw her she started to take ascorbic acid 2 g t.i.d., niacin 0.5 g t.i.d., l-lysine for herpes 250 mg t.i.d., zinc sulfate 220 mg od, pyridoxine 250 mg od, and

TABLE 24
Number of Patients with Cancer of the Cervix, Uterus, and Ovary Surviving up to Five Years

Patients Alive By Years							
	N	1	2	3	4	5	Alive
Cervix	7	6	5	5	3		5, range 3 - 12
Uterus	13	9	9	7	5	4	7, range 3 - 12
Ovary	24	15	10	5	4	3	6, range 3 - 11
Ovary-control	Out of 11, 9 died the first year, two in the second year.						

selenium 200 mcg od. She was not able to tolerate niacin and this was changed to niacinamide. By March 1984 she was free of genital herpes. In March 1988 she was normal and was still well in September 1996.

(2) Case #41
Born in 1946, she was first seen in August 1984. In May 1984, following a positive cone biopsy for cancer, she was advised to have an hysterectomy, but she refused. After I saw her she began to take ascorbic acid 4 g t.i.d., niacinamide 0.5 g t.i.d., vitamin E 400 iu od, and selenium 200 mcg od. Early in 1985 she did have her hysterectomy. She was alive and well in September 1996.

(3) Case #224
Born in 1914, she was first seen (for cancer) in August 1987.

This patient first came to see me in 1985 for a variety of physical complaints, for which I started her on linodil (inositol niacinate) 3 grams per day and ascorbic acid 3 grams per day. In November 1986 she was infected with candida and was started on mycostatin. In July 1987 she noted that she was bleeding after voiding and on July 21 received a hysterectomy for cancer, diagnosed as Stage I endometrial adenocanthoma. I modified her program to include ascorbic acid 4 g t.i.d., linodil 2 g t.i.d., and vitamin K 5 mg od.

She reported 2 November 1987 that she had completed a series of radiation treatments. She was depressed at that time, and I therefore started her on Elavil 25 mg hs. In December 1987 her mood was good, she was no longer depressed. I added vitamin K 10 mg per day to her program and zinc chelate 30 mg per day. Her last cancer check up had been clear.

In June 1988 she reported she was on ascorbic acid 6 g per day, linodil 3 g per day, thyroid 60 mg od, mycostatin 1 million units t.i.d., folic acid 5 mg od, vitamin K 5 mg b.i.d., and selenium 200 mcg b.i.d. She was doing well. In June 1991 she was still doing very well and had had no recurrence of her cancer. She was still normal in September 1996.

Patients with Ovarian Cancer Surviving 7 or More Years

Out of 26 cases of ovarian cancer, 6 are alive for an average of 5.5 years, range 2 to 10. None of the controls survived the first year. Three patients lived over 7 years. Their brief histories are given below.

(1) Case #23

Born in 1941, she was first seen in May 1982. Early in 1981 both ovaries were removed. She was then started on chemotherapy, adriamyacin and cisplatinate, but treatment had to be stopped prematurely because her white cell count dropped too far. She had her last treatment in January. Following that she received radiation for six weeks. A laparotomy later that year showed there had been a recurrence. I advised her to take ascorbic acid 4 g t.i.d., niacinamide 0.5 g t.i.d., pyridoxine 250 mg od, zinc sulfate 220 mg od, selenium 200 micrograms od, and vitamin A 50,000 iu od. One month later she had reduced her ascorbic acid to 2 g daily, but by the end of the year she had been averaging 3 g od.

On 10 April 1984 she was found to have secondaries in her bones. She increased her ascorbic acid to 12 g o d and the selenium to 400 mcg. On 25 April 1985 she had further surgery, followed by 20 more radiations. By then she had a secondary carcinoma in the cerebellum causing severe headaches. On 7 April 1988 she was normal. She had remained on her vitamin regimen only until the end of November 1985. After ten years she was still well and follow-up was discontinued.

(2) Case #197

Born in 1918, she was first seen in February 1989. In May 1985 both ovaries and the uterus were removed with cancer of the ovaries. After that she was given 3 sessions of chemotherapy and 32 sessions of radiation. Her attitude was positive. She watched her diet, exercised, and was active in a hope group. She was advised to start on calcium ascorbate 2 g t.i.d., niacinamide 0.5 g t.i.d., selenium 200 mcg b.i.d., beta carotene 10,000 iu per day, B-complex 50 mg od, and zinc citrate 50 mg od.

In September 1989 she was clear of cancer and still on her megavitamin program. In July 1991 she was still clear and was discharged from the cancer clinic. On 31 December 1991 she remained normal, free of any cancer, but she was developing a cataract in her eye. I added riboflavin 100 mg to her daily program. On November 1992 she was told by her ophthalmologist that there had been no further deterioration in her vision. She told me she was able to see better than before. Her mood was good. On 2 March 1993 she was still free of cancer, as she was on 3 September 1993 and 11 April 1994. Her only complaint was severe arthritis which had come on over the previous two months. She was still well in her seventies on September 1996.

(3) Case #298
Born in 1926, she was first seen in January 1989. After suffering fatigue for a long time, she was admitted for investigation in January 1988. An ovarian cyst the size of a grapefruit was removed. Following that she had 5 chemotherapy sessions and 6 weeks of daily radiation. At the end she was very tired but she began to recover slowly. I advised her to take ascorbic acid 12 g, niacinamide 1.5, beta carotene 20,000 iu, and selenium 600 mcg daily. In February 1989 she told me she had to decrease the amount of ascorbic acid because it caused heartburn. On 31 December 1993 she was suffering from fibromyalgia, chronic fatigue syndrome, and arthritic pains, but there had been no recurrence of her cancer. She was on ascorbic acid 3 g daily. She had discontinued the rest of the vitamin program but stated she was going to resume the whole program. She was still free of cancer in September 1996.

– Abram Hoffer

Sarcoma and Melanoma

Summary

Osteogenic sarcoma is the most common malignant tumor of bone and may be primary or secondary as a complication of other bone disease. Primary osteogenic sarcoma occurs more commonly in people under age 20 and peaks during their teens. Males get it twice as often. The most common location is around the knee in the femur in the most rapidly growing part of the bone. Bone forming cells release alkaline phosophatases and these are elevated in the blood. As usual the causes are not known but they do include irradiation. It was once described as an occupational cancer in workers exposed to radium. With amputation alone, the 5 year survival was 20 percent, with death caused by lung metastases. Modern treatment has improved, using a combination of reconstructive surgery, chemotherapy, and radiation; amputation is no longer inevitable as it was in 1960. Ewings sarcoma occurs in a younger age group in the extremities and has about a 75 percent survival using all three standard modalities of treatment. The survival rate was 5 percent when only surgery was used. The main symptoms are pain and a mass.

Secondary osteosarcomas represent about 80 percent of all sarcomas. They are secondary to previous bone disease ,including cysts and Pagets disease, and peak over age 40.

Sarcomas are rather rare. Out of 1,060 patients in my series with cancer, only eight were sarcomas.

Case Histories

Of 3 sarcoma patients, one is alive 3 years, the second lived 9 years and died of a coronary at age 80, and the third is still alive after more than 10 years. Twelve patients received total treatment for melanoma. Four died the first year. Three died in the second year, and 5 are still alive over 2 years. All the 6 controls died the first year.

(1) Case #6

Born in 1908, he was first seen in January 1980. During March 1978 he began to feel a stabbing pain in his left groin. Early in 1979 this was traced to a cancer in his pelvic bone. It was spindle cell sarcoma (neurofibrosarcoma) which was spreading internally. Surgery relieved the pain, but later he was given radiation, completing the series in April. By the end of the year the mass had started growing again. More radiation was not recommended, and he rejected chemotherapy. He was also under severe stress because his wife was dying from cancer. After her death he told his physician that he had nothing much left to live for, that he intended to go to a clinic in Mexico even if it meant blowing his entire estate. I advised him to start on ascorbic acid 4 g t.i.d., niacinamide 0.5 g t.i.d., pyridoxine 250 mg od, zinc gluconate 100 mg od, and a mineral preparation.

A month later he told me he could not tolerate more than 12 g of ascorbic acid daily. I recommended to his referring physician that he give him sodium ascorbate intravenously 2.5 g, 3 times per week. But in that first month a chronic boil (staph) under the tumor on his left leg had healed, he had no edema, and his mood was normal. The radiologist reported in 2

May 1980, "Comparison is made with the previous study of February 7, 1979, which showed an apparent expanding destructional lesion involving the superior ramus of the left pubic bone which was involved with Pagets disease compatible with sarcomatous change of Pagets. Present study shows marked improvement with some apparent bony reconstruction and the left superior pubic ramus. There has certainly been no further bony destruction in the interior." On 4 September 1980 his physician gave him his last injection. In March 1986 he had a small basal cell carcinoma of the skin on his nose treated. He remained well until he died in August 1989 from a coronary.

(2) Case #22
Born in 1965, she was first seen in August 1981. In October 1979 she developed pain in her left shoulder. The deltoid muscle was enlarged and tender and overlaid a broad-based mass which involved the upper third of the humerus and was several centimeters thick. An x-ray showed the upper half of the humerus was abnormal. The lesion involved the entire cortex and medullary canal along with onion skinning. There was also a soft tissue mass in the deltoid region. She was diagnosed with Ewings sarcoma and given chemotherapy and radiotherapy for two years. In July 1981 residual tumor was still present. On 26 August 1981 I advised her to take ascorbic acid 12 g, niacinamide 3.0 g, pyridoxine 250 mg, zinc gluconate 100 mg, and dolomite 4 tablets, all daily.

In July 1984 she suffered a fracture of the humerus. Early in 1984 she had surgery to fill in the bone. In July 1985 she was well and was working. In 1989 she had a child. At 10-year follow-up she was well.

(3) Case #495
Born in 1957, he was first seen in June 1993. In 1981 he had a large liposarcoma removed from his leg. At first the surgeon thought the leg would have to be amputated. The mass was 10 by 5 cm large. After that he was given 30 irradiation sessions. He was well until three months before he saw me. By then he had another large mass in his abdomen which he could palpate. It was adherent to the peritoneum. The mass was removed and he was told he had a 25 percent chance it would not recur. He started himself on a good

multivitamin program. I advised him to take ascorbic acid 12 g, B-complex 50s, niacinamide 1.5 g, beta carotene 50,000 iu, vitamin E 2,000 iu, selenium 300 mcg, zinc citrate 50 mg, and folic acid 15 mg, all daily. He was still well in September 1996.

– Abram Hoffer

5 CONTROVERSY

The Cancer Industry and Orthomolecular Medicine

Orthomolecular medicine, especially the optimum intake of vitamins and other nutrients, may have its greatest value in improving general health, potentiating the body's natural protective mechanism and decreasing the incidence of all disease. However, practitioners of conventional medicine have in the past been more interested in the treatment of disease than in the prevention of disease. The lack of interest in preventive medicine may be the main reason for the slow rate of incorporation of orthomolecular medicine into conventional medicine. Another reason is the bias against vitamins as prophylactic and therapeutic agents, except for controlling their own deficiency diseases.

We hold the medical authorities, by their failure to make proper assessments of the evidence, responsible for this state of affairs among practicing physicians. The practicing physician is usually forced by circumstances to accept the statements of the medical authorities. By their control of the sources of funds for support of research, the medical authorities are able to prevent substantiating studies from being carried out. In 1973 the officers of the National Cancer Institute refused to take any action to check the observations made by Dr Ewan Cameron on the value of megadoses of vitamin C for patients with advanced cancer. They said that it would be necessary first for animal studies to be carried out, but then for 10 years rejected applications for grants to carry out animal studies, and ignored the positive results of the animal studies when they finally were carried out. Almost 20 years later in 1990, the National Cancer Institute at last took a serious interest in the possibility that vitamin C may have significant value in the treatment of cancer, as well as in cancer prevention. At the same time, the American Cancer Society changed from describing the use of vitamins to help to control cancer as "quackery" to advocating a high intake of vitamin C for the control of cancer, though the Society recommends that the high intake be obtained by selecting foods rich in this vitamin. The Society seems to feel that there is something improper about taking advantage of the series of great discoveries made early in this century that led to the availability of vitamin C tablets at low cost which can provide more of the vitamin than can be derived from foods, giving even more protection.

There is a political context for this state of medical research into the efficacy of vitamin C for preventing and treating cancer. A thorough analysis of the so-called vitamin C and cancer controversy has been made by Dr Evelleen Richards in her book *Vitamin C and Cancer: Medicine or Politics.* While reviewing the work of Dr Ewan Cameron and Linus Pauling reported in their book Cancer and Vitamin C, she points out that Dr Cameron "was quite well known professionally in Scottish surgical and cancer circles, and had established a reputation as offering some promising theoretical insights into the cancer process.... Cameron's work was certainly not viewed as deviant or unorthodox." When he began to give megadoses of vitamin C to patients, however, the situation changed: "From the beginning of their collaborative clinical research, Pauling and Cameron experienced all the difficulties and frustrations Cameron had anticipated, of convincing his 'incredulous' profession that such a common place and innocuous substance as vitamin C might have anything to offer cancer patients. Their presentation problems were compounded by the radical differences between their therapeutic approach and that of conventional oncologists."

These differences include, of course, a difference in attitude towards the toxicity and disagreeable side effects of conventional therapies, a difference in opinion about the amount of detailed supervision required by the oncologist, a difference in opinion about the ease of access of the patient to the vitamin or drug, and a difference attitude about the cost of treatments. Although patients are always supposed to be able to accept or reject a suggested treatment, it is clear that they have more control over their own lives with orthomolecular medicine than with conventional medicine. Many patients, dissatisfied with the results of conventional treatment, search for help from the unconventional forms of cancer treatment. It is hard for them to get advice on this point: most oncologists and other physicians simply say that none of the unconventional therapies has any value – they are all quackery. Dr Richards concludes that "the history of the vitamin C and cancer controversy is best understood as a political struggle concerning control over the determination and evaluation of cancer treatments."

Among the various attempts to suppress or discredit research studies showing the efficacy of vitamin C, a study led by C.G. Moertel at The Mayo Clinic, published in 1985 in *The New England Journal of Medicine*, provides a good example of how the cancer establishment works. Every physician seems to know about this study, at least enough to say to the patient, 'The Mayo Clinic showed that vitamin C has no value against cancer.' This statement is false, however, because the study was so flawed as to make it quite unreliable. In this study, 50 patients with advanced colorectal cancer were given vitamin C, 10 g per day. They were given the vitamin for a median time of only 75 days. During this first 75 days only one patient died. After being taken off vitamin C, the patients then began to die rapidly, about half of them dying during the next 75 days. We had previously pointed out that there is a potential rebound effect when high-dose vitamin C is suddenly stopped, and that it might be dangerous for cancer patients to do so. (We repeat the recommendation that the intake of high doses of vitamin C and other nutrients not be suddenly stopped.) If a detailed analysis of the Mayo Clinic case histories were to be made, it might provide valuable information about how serious the rebound effect is for cancer patients, but Dr Moertel refused to release information about the investigation other than that in the published paper. In their paper the Mayo Clinic investigators ask why Cameron observed a very large effect of vitamin C in extending the survival times of cancer patients, whereas they had observed no such effect, but rather some decrease in life expectancy. The obvious answer, that Cameron's patients continued to receive the vitamin for years but their patients for only a median of 75 days, is not given in their paper. Careful reading of their paper is required to discover the statement, in fine print, that the vitamin C was stopped after the median times of 75 days; in fact, Dr. Cameron himself read the papers with great interest after it was published without noticing that there was this astonishing difference between the Mayo Clinic treatment and his treatment. The claim made by the Mayo Clinic investigators that they were repeating Cameron's work is accordingly not true. It is this claim that has led most physicians to believe that vitamin C had no value in controlling cancer.

Many other misleading reports of trials of unconventional methods of treating cancer and other diseases with vitamins or other unorthodox therapies have also been published. An example is study led by R.G. Knodell that claimed that they were repeating the work of F. Morishige and A. Murata on the value of vitamin C in protecting against viral hepatitis in surgical patients who had received transfusions of blood. Knodell reported that they had found no protection, whereas Morishige and Murata had reported almost complete protection. Elsewhere, we have pointed out that Morishige and Murata had given a median of 10 g of vitamin C per day for usually 6 months to their patients, whereas Knodell et al, had given only 3 g per day for only 16 days. This difference in the treatment is so great that it is misleading to claim that Knodell et al. had shown vitamin C to be ineffective in controlling post transfusion hepatitis.

Beyond these methodologically flawed attempts to discredit the value of vitamin C, there is a fundamental resistance within the medical establishment to even consider any alternative form of treatment, especially nutritional treatment.

In *Cancer and Vitamin C*, Cameron and Pauling express an opinion about four unconventional cancer therapies on the basis of the available evidence. They conclude that the Max Gerson treatment of eating raw fruits and vegetables and drinking large amounts of fruit and vegetable juices, which provide large amounts of vitamins and minerals, has considerable value. The Coley treatment, use of mixed toxins to stimulate the immune system, probably also was beneficial for some patients. They were unable to form a reliable opinion about either Laitrile or Krebiozin. Their opinion of vitamin C was, of course, a good one.

Unorthodox methods of controlling cancer have been discussed in many other books and articles, most notably *The Cancer Industry: Unraveling the Politics* by Ralph Moss. Moss gives a good brief discussion of Mayo Clinic study, showing its "clear intention of blowing the vitamin-C-and-cancer controversy off the medical map." He also provides good discussions of many other alternative cancer treatments, noting that the advocates of many of these treatments have just as good medical credentials as their opponents.

Moss also asks if there really is a "cancer establishment," and while answering that there is no such organized body, nevertheless notes, "the leaders of the top organizations discussed in this book are certainly familiar with each other and interlock on many committees, panels, and boards. Sometimes they are friendly, and sometimes they disagree. What holds them together, however, is a community of interests and ideas. The top leaders generally see eye-to-eye on the major questions concerning cancer. They favor cure over prevention. They emphasize the use of patentable and/or synthetic chemicals over readily available or natural methods. They set the trends in research, and are careful to stay within the bounds of what is acceptable and fashionable at the moment." Moss concludes, "it is the system itself, rather than any particular clique of individuals, which is really to blame for failure to make progress against the cancer problem. In particular, the fact that cancer management is itself a big business means that it must function according to the rules of profit-oriented institutions."

– Linus Pauling

Difficulties Faced by Patients

As a result of this controversy, many of the patients I treated underwent this added ordeal of gaining the confidence of their family, friends, and medical practitioners in the orthomolecular program.

1. **Medical Skeptism**: Usually physicians treating a patient are supportive; when an oncologist recommends chemotherapy, the referring physician will support this. When a depressed patient is started on antidepressants, this is supported by the referring doctor. Physicians usually will not downgrade a treatment recommended by the specialist to whom they have referred the patient.

Cancer patients receiving orthomolecular treatment often did not get this kind of support, however. At most, physicians felt that the treatment would do no harm, but it could do no good because it was simply an elaborate placebo. Because of the reluctance of physicians to accept the validity of orthomolecular medicine, patients lost valuable time while they were being treated with standard therapy. One of the major criticisms of complementary medicine (conventional plus orthomolecular) is that it denies or delays the use of standard treatment. I think that this argument is not based on fact for nearly every patient. In my experience, patients seeking complementary medicine have already been treated by conventional methods, usually unsuccessfully. Failures provide the main reservoir of patients seeking help outside the medical profession. Even if it were true, there is little proof that for most cancers standard treatment prolongs life or even improves its quality. What does a woman gain when she has a mastectomy followed by irradiation or chemotherapy, with all the attendant pain and discomfort, if all she can expect is more discomfort for a few months? The pain and discomfort become much less of a problem if many more years of high quality life can be achieved. For many types of cancer, the wisest course may be no standard treatment until it can be shown that the outcome is much better than it is now. I do not think that the criticism is well thought out, which may be why so many patients seek complementary treatment and even alternative treatments.

Treatment should be started as early as possible. This includes orthomolecular treatment. As soon as the diagnosis has been established, the entire comprehensive treatment program should be started. There is no clash between using nutrition and supplements and accepting surgery, irradiation, or chemotherapy. In this series of 134 patients only two patients started the entire comprehensive program as soon as the diagnosis was established. One was a family friend, the other a relative. Normally patients referred to me have to wait several months before they can be seen, unless the referring physician tells me they are an emergency. I see emergencies within three days of the referral being received. Each cancer patient was considered an emergency and was seen within three to four days, if I was informed they had cancer. A few were seen after the usual waiting period, and I discovered they had cancer only during the first interview.

Negative publicity, which appeared regularly in the media, was not a factor. It had already been discounted by the patients who decided to seek referral to me. Patients who respect this type of uninformed, negative information do not seek additional treatment. If the standard treatment fails, they accept the dying role and need only palliative treatment for pain or depression. It would help, however, if the disseminators of public information were less certain, less dogmatic about the uses of nutrition and nutrients, so that patients now wavering in their decision to seek orthomolecular help would come earlier in the treatment process. Fortunately, there has been a significant change in the attitude of the media and many more favorable stories about the beneficial properties of vitamins and vitamin supplements are now reported almost on a weekly basis.

2. **Family Hostility**: Family hostility was rare, but in a few cases the family believed the patients were wasting money on useless treatment. They had heard so much about quackery that they could not believe that the orthomolecular approach could help. Spouses usually were very helpful and were always involved in the program. Naturally, spouses who objected strenuously would have prevented cancer patients from being referred.

3. **Cancer Clinic Hostility**: The hostility of the Cancer Clinic apparently did not deter patients. Generally, I saw failures who were annoyed or angry with the Clinic. Several threatened to sue the Clinic, but did not. When patients told their oncologists they were taking orthomolecular therapy, they were, at first, advised to stop the program, for, they said, it was useless and could be toxic. Chemotherapists were especially insistent that the vitamins would prevent the chemotherapy from working. The Clinic nutritionists usually gave the patients incorrect advice – for example, that vitamin C would cause kidney stones. Over the past few years the oncologists have become more neutral and will make fewer negative statements without making any supportive ones.

The Clinic showed its antagonism in other ways. For the first 10 years they were very reluctant to send me copies of their clinical case records. I was entitled to them since they were also my patients and legally they could not have refused. Patients always gave their consent for me to see their files. However, since then there has been no problem.

4. **False Information**: A patient I had placed on selenium 600 micrograms per day was advised by the clerk in a health food store that this dosage would kill her. In the same way, many years ago druggists would advise my patients that vitamin C would cause kidney stones. This type of advice has, however, now become very infrequent. A fairly common problem is for druggists to confuse niacin and niacinamide. More recently, health food stores have been offering advice about the treatment of cancer which has been contradictory. I would prefer if they would not hand out their advice so freely.

5. **Insurance Agencies**: In British Columbia, all residents are entitled to reimbursement for prescription drugs. The amount varies from 80 percent over and above a certain deductible amount, to almost 100 percent for people over 65, and to 100 percent for all patients receiving social assistance. Of the nutrients, only niacin and folic acid are considered prescription drugs. Other anti-cancer agents are covered, irrespective of cost, and even when there is little evidence they are even palliative.

6. **Specialization**: Another problem arose because I did not see these patients often enough. Most of them had no major psychiatric disease. It would have been difficult to continue to see them, as I am a psychiatrist. Reviewing these patients, I have concluded that they should have been seen more often in order to provide encouragement and to answer questions. Many patients I had not seen for several years had gone off their regimen months or years before they suffered a recurrence. Had I been seeing them regularly they might have stayed on the program. Of course, the general practitioner should have helped their patients maintain their program, but in many cases these patients would not have seen any doctor.

– Abram Hoffer

Paradigm Shift

Despite the machinations of the cancer establishment or industry, we believe that this control will soon come to an end. The value of high-dose vitamin C and other nutrients in the prevention and treatment of cancer is so striking that it can no longer be neglected. During the next decade we should see an astonishing decrease in the incidence of and mortality from cancer and also other diseases, as the value of these remarkable substances becomes generally recognized.

– Linus Pauling

Historically, such changes in attitude or view or 'paradigm' within scientific thinking take about 40 years from being first proven to being widely accepted as historians like Thomas Kuhn in his Structure of Scientific Revolutions have shown. The resistance to new ideas is formidable, as Dr Pauling discovered when he published his classical 1969 report in Science entitled "Orthomolecular Psychiatry." He was astonished by the vehemence of the attack on his views and even on his sanity, led by the leaders of the American Psychiatric Association. In our research studies on the value of vitamin B-3 for treating heart disease and schizophrenia, Dr Humphry Osmond and I received similar attacks, which are documented in my Vitamin B-3 and Schizophrenia: Discovery, Recovery, Controversy.

Medical science has not yet developed a system which will examine the value of new treatments if they are within a new paradigm. I define a new treatment as one which crosses from an old established paradigm into a new one and helps to move medicine into the new one. Thus, after the use of antibiotics was established, the development of new antibiotics does not constitute a new treatment. It is merely an expansion of the older treatment already in general use. It may be better, more efficient, less toxic but it is not new. This is why the introduction of new antibiotics does not generate any controversy in the profession. The introduction of the steroid hormones for the treatment of arthritis was a new paradigm, but the use of different types of steroid hormones does not constitute a new treatment. The use of new variants of psychotherapy does not mean we have new treatment. They are merely variations on a theme and often random ones which depend almost entirely on the idiosyncrasies of the inventor of these forms of psychotherapy. There are 200 forms of psychotherapy which have been described over the years.

The introduction of the vitamin deficiency paradigm required many years of hard work on the part of the original innovators before it became generally accepted. Once this had been accepted, it required very little effort to use vitamins for new deficiency disease, but these are not new, merely variations. The use of megadoses of vitamins was a new paradigm and stoutly resisted. My colleagues and I published our report that niacin lowered cholesterol levels in 1955, but only about 35 years later did niacin achieve world-wide acclaim as one of the best substances for doing so. It is still not widely used since it cannot compete in advertising with the major drugs used today. It is an orphan compound. The other drugs have their mighty protective parents who fight for them with tooth and nail.

The use of new drugs for chemotherapy is not controversial. They are merely variations on the same theme, but the introduction of nutrients as treatment is a brand new paradigm and is still stoutly resisted. Once one vitamin is accepted as having therapeutic properties, it will not be difficult to introduce other vitamins because the new paradigm will have been accepted.

For these reasons I think today that the orthomolecular treatment for cancer will not be established by the year 2000. It will probably take another 20 years. The costs to society will be incalculable.

There is a method which would speed up the examination of new treatments to show either that they are effective or not effective, but it would require a major shift in public and medical attitude toward new discovery. In other words, it would require a new paradigm. This method would proceed as follows.

First, governments would create one or more clinical medical investigative units. These would be staffed by physicians who have had experience in clinical trials – all clinical trials, including the usual open clinical models on to some of the controlled comparative studies. These physicians would not be allowed to have cross appointments with any other institutions, including medical associations, hospitals, universities, medical schools, drug companies, and other government departments. This is to prevent the heavy hand of conservatism from deadening the investigative spirit of the institution. This unique institute would report directly to the legislature.

Second, whenever a physician or scientist published a paper where it is claimed that a certain treatment had been used and found successful this would be immediately examined by the institution. The difficulty in getting these reports published would be the first barrier the physician claiming a new treatment would have to cross. The institution, after having examined the report, would immediately send an on site investigator to visit the physician making these claims and would examine the records and, even more important, would examine the patients of these physicians who had been treated. If the claims were confirmed – i.e., patients said to be well are well – the study would enter its second phase.

The original physician would be invited to join the staff at the institution for a period of time and would be paid for his loss of income because of leaving the practice. At the institution the physician would be allowed to treat a series of patients using his methods, but watching him would be some of the clinical staff of the institution who would be there in order to see what he was doing and to become familiar with the method. Once the physician was satisfied that the investigative team were familiar with his method and he had confidence that they would use his treatment as he would have, he would return home and the third phase of the investigation would start.

The investigative team would then test a series of patients using exactly the same treatment as they had been taught by the original physician. After a period of time that would be acceptable to the original physician, they would evaluate the results of the treatment. They would then prepare a report which would describe what they had done and would finally divide the patients in main categories such as well, much improved, not improved, and so on. The report would not provide any opinions on the worth of the treatment. The report would be presented to the legislature and published as an objective statement of what the investigative team had observed.

Physicians everywhere could then read the report and decide on their own whether or not they wished to use the new treatment. They would not have to depend upon the opinions of professors in medical schools or in the leading institutions. If this approach had been used when my colleagues and I first reported that niacin lowered cholesterol, it would have become used generally within about five years instead of 35.

If this or a similar attitude towards scientific research into health problems were to be adopted by the medical establishment, not only would research be able to proceed beyond the shibboleth of the double-blind standard, but, most importantly, the lives of many more patients suffering from cancer and other serious disease would be prolonged, improved, and saved.

In sum, our research has shown that every cancer patient should give serious consideration to accepting appropriate conventional therapy, after being given evidence that it is appropriate to the case, and that every cancer patient, starting as early as possible, should follow the regimen of nutrients described in this book, preferably under the supervision of a physician who practices orthomolecular medicine.

– Abram Hoffer

APPENDICES

APPENDIX 1

Hardin Jones Biostatistical Analysis of Mortality Data for Cohorts of Cancer Patients

This appendix consists of the detailed biostatistical analysis of the survival times of the original series of 134 patients. Some of their case histories have already been presented, and some of the results of the analysis have previously been discussed. The paper was written by Linus Pauling and Abram Hoffer and first published in the August 1990 issue of the Journal of Orthomolecular Medicine and then reprinted in the 1993 edition of Cancer and Vitamin C by Ewan Cameron and Linus Pauling.

One of us has recently pointed out (Pauling, 1989) that the biostatistical analysis of mortality data for a cohort of cancer patients is made more powerful by the use of the principle discovered by Hardin Jones in 1956, and this principle has been applied in the formulation of a set of criteria for the validity of clinical test of a treatment of cancer patients (Pauling & Herman, 1989). A important reason for carrying out such a test is the determination of the mean survival times of the homogeneous subcohorts that compose the cohort being tested. The problem of separating the cohort into homogeneous subcohorts and evaluating their mean survival times for a test in which most of the patient have died by the termination date has been discussed (Pauling, 1989); we now attack the problem for the case of survival of a large fraction of the patients.

Analysis of Mortality Data for a Homogeneous Cohort

Hardin Jones reported (1956) that published mortality data for cohorts of similar cancer patients indicate the death rate to be constant:

$$- \frac{dN}{dt} = \alpha N_o \quad (1)$$

$$N = N_o e \cdot \alpha t \quad (2)$$

Here N_o is the number of patients entering the study at time t = 0, N is the number surviving at time t, and α is the death rate.

The fraction surviving at time t, S, is given by the equation

$$S = N/N_o = e \cdot \alpha t \quad (3)$$

The plot of ln S vs t is a straight line with slope $\cdot \alpha$. The value of the mean survival time τ is α^{-1}. One of us (Pauling) has pointed out that there are many ways to calculate r for a homogeneous cohort. The approximate equality of the values of τ obtained in several ways is a useful test of homogeneity, supplementing inspection of the Hardin Jones plot to check for upward curvature of the ln S line.

For a homogeneous cohort the value of τ for N survivors is α^{-1} (Equation 3). Another way of evaluating τ results from the fact that the mean survival time of all N_o patients is τ and the mean additional survival time of the N survivors is also τ. Let $<\tau>$ be the survival time of the N_o - N patients who have died and $<\tau^+>$ be that of the N survivors (who may have entered the study at any time). The sum of the total survival times can be written in two ways, which must be equal:

$$N_o\tau = (N_o \cdot N) <t> + N<\tau^+> + N\tau \quad (4)$$

The last term expresses the fact that the N survivors have remaining mean survival time τ. From this equation we obtain another expression for τ.

$$\tau = (\Sigma t + \Sigma t^{+}) / (N_o - N) \qquad (5)$$

This equation is unreliable when $N_O - N$ is small.

Motivation for the Formulation of the Method of Biostatistical Analysis Based on the Hardin Jones Principle

One of us (Hoffer) is a biochemist and psychiatrist who, about 40 years ago (in collaboration with Humphry Osmond) began treating schizophrenic patients with very large daily intakes of vitamin B3 (nicotinic acid or nicotinamide) and other vitamins, including ascorbic acid. He and his collaborators in 1957 reported the results of the first randomized double-blind study made in the field of psychiatry (Hoffer et al., 1957). He also observed that a few mentally ill patients who also suffered from cancer seemed to gain some control over this disease while being given psychiatric treatment by him. He began a controlled study in July 1978 (patient No. 84, cancer of the pancreas). Between that date and April 15, 1988, 134 patients with cancer were accepted by him (column A in Tables 1, 2, 4 and 5). Survival times are given to the termination date of the study, January 1, 1990.

About 25% of the patients rejected the ascorbic acid and also the other vitamins. The others received from 3 to 40 g of vitamin C per day, taken by mouth, mostly 12 g per day. It soon became evident that the vitamin C patients survived much longer than the others, and an effort was made to evaluate the mean survival times by the conventional methods of biostatistical analysis. This effort was not very successful, in that these methods do not give proper consideration to the survivors, those patients still alive at the termination of the study, who comprise about 50% of the vitamin C patients. It was then recognized that the acceptance of the Hardin Jones principle permitted the formulation of a more powerful method of biostatistical analysis of mortality data for cohorts of cancer patients. Some results of applying this method have been reported (Pauling, 1989; Pauling & Herman, 1989). We now report on its application to cohorts with a large number of survivors at the termination of a study, with the 134 patients as an example. To decrease the effect of statistical fluctuations we have combined female patients with cancer of the breast, ovary, uterus, cervix and fallopian tube into two cohorts (receiving vitamins and not receiving vitamins) and the remaining patients, both male and female, with cancer of the colon, lung, prostate, pancreas, and others, into another two cohorts.

Analysis of Survival Times Listed in Tables 1 and 2

Separate analyses of the mean survival times for Table I and Table 2 show that they are nearly equal; hence they can be combined, to give somewhat increased reliability to the average value of the mean survival time τ. Moreover, the analysis indicates some heterogeneity, as might be expected from the many different kinds of cancer represented. It is found, however, that the only resolution into subcohorts that can be achieved is to a large subcohort of 31 patients, with $\tau = 5.7 \pm 0.4$ mo (Table 3), and a small subcohort of 2 patients, with τ about 48 mo. The small subcohort consists of No. 14, with $\tau = 45$ mo(cancer of the testis), and No. 31, with $\tau^{+} = 49+$ mo (cancer of the fallopian tube,). The probability that either of these is a member of the main subcohort is less than 1 %. Neither of these two kinds of cancer is represented in Tables 4 and 5.

Biostatistical Treatment of Cohorts With Many Survivors

The analysis of mortality data for a cohort with many survivors is more difficult than that for a cohort with few survivors, especially if the cohort is heterogeneous; it is, however, possible to carry out such an analysis by application of the Hardin Jones principle. For a homogeneous cohort the value of T given by Equation 5 is reliable if a good number of patients have died. Another equation can be obtained by discussing the values of the square of the survival time. For a homogeneous cohort the following equation is valid (Pauling, 1980):

$$\{\langle t^2 \rangle / 2\}^{1/2} = \tau \qquad (6)$$

$$\text{or } \langle t^2 \rangle = 2\,\tau^2 \qquad (7)$$

TABLE 1

Values of survival times for 11 female patients with cancer of the breast, ovary, uterus, or fallopian tube who had not received ascorbic acid or other vitamins as an adjunct to other therapy (column 7). Column A gives the date when the patient was first seen by A.H. and entered into this study. Column B gives the number of months between the diagnosis of cancer and the date in column A. The date of death or the state of health on January 1, 1990 is given in column C.

		A	Age	Type	B	Treat-ment[a]	C	Survival (mo)
4.	M.B.	09/81	37	Ovary	9	R,C	Died 0 1 /82	2.6
7	J.C.	01/80	57	Breast	3	S,C	Died 04/80	3.7
9.	A.A.	07/84	38	Ovary	3	S,C	Died 07/85	12
31.	E.H.	11/85	50	Fallopian tube	2	S	Ill	49+
59.	J.M.	10/86	30	Breast	21	S,R,C	Died 03/87	6
65.	D.P.	06/85	64	Ovary	12	S,C	Died 09/85	3.2
76.	M.S.	12/81	56	Uterus	32	S,C	Died 03/82	4.0
79.	N.T.	11/80	65	Breast	36	S	Died 0 1 /81	1.8
81.	S.W.	08/82	53	Breast	48	S,C	Died 10/82	2.2
113.	J.G.	07/87	77	Ovary	7	S,C	Died 11/87	4.0
115.	S.A.	06/86	57	Breast	12	S,C,R	Died 10/86	4.2

[a] S = surgery, R = radiation, C = chemotherapy, N = no treatment

With t_i^+ the survival time of the ith patient at the termination date of the study, we write for the predicted total survival time t_i the relation

$$t_i = t_i^+ \delta_i \tag{8}$$

The mean value of δ_i is τ. The value of t_i^2 is

$$t_i^2 = (t_i^+ + \delta_i)^2 = (t_i^+)^2 + 2\delta_i t_i^+ + \delta_i^2 \tag{9}$$

and for N_0 members of the cohort with N survivors Equation 7 becomes

$$2N_0 t^2 = \Sigma(t^+)^2 + 2\Sigma\delta_i t_i^+ + 2N\tau^2 \tag{10}$$

TABLE 3
Values of the mean survival time t calculated by 4 methods for the cohort of 31 patients in Tables 1 and 2 (No. 14 and No. 31 not included, see text).

Method	τ(mo)
$1.781 \exp < \ln t >$	6.2
$\{<t^{1/2}> / \Gamma(3/2)\}^2$	5.6
$<t>$	6.0
$\{<t^2>/2\}^{1/2}$	5.0
Mean	5.7
Mean deviation	0.4

In this equation $\Sigma\delta_i^2$ has been replaced by $2\tau^2$, because the values of δ_i have the distribution given by Equation 2. Moreover, since the values of δ_i are not correlated with those of t_i^+, δ_i can be moved to the left of the summation sign and replaced by its mean value τ, giving the equation

$$2\,(N_o - N)\,\tau^2 = \Sigma t^2 + \Sigma(t^+)^2 + 2\tau\,\Sigma t^+ \qquad (11)$$

Solution of this quadratic equation gives

$$\tau = \Sigma t^+/2(N_o - N) \pm [\{\Sigma t^2 + \Sigma(t^+)^2\}/2(N_o \cdot N) - <t^+>^2/4]^{1/2} \qquad (12)$$

Other ways of evaluating τ for a homogeneous cohort with no survivors might be adapted to the case of a homogeneous cohort with many survivors by changing t_i^+ to t_i, Equation 8, but we have not found any good analytical way of doing this.

Resolving a Cohort into Two Homogeneous Subcohorts

Let f_1 be the fraction of the first subcohort, with mean survival time τ_1, and f_2 (equal to $1 - f_1$) that of the second subcohort, with mean survival time τ_2 larger than τ_1. The mean values $<\tau>$ from Equation 5 and $<\tau^2>^{1/2}$ from Equation 12 permit two of the three unknowns to be evaluated if the third is known. We have the relations

$$<\tau> = f_1\tau_1 + f_2\tau_2 \qquad (13)$$
$$\text{and } <\tau^2> = f_1\tau_1^2 + f_2\tau_2^2 \qquad (14)$$

Let $< \Leftrightarrow > = <\tau>$ and $q = <\tau^2>$. A lower limit for τ_2 is given by the equation

$$\tau_2 > q/\Leftrightarrow \qquad (15)$$

and an upper limit to f_2 by the equation

$$f_2 < \Leftrightarrow^2/q \qquad (16)$$

If τ_2 is known, then τ_1 and f_1 are given by the equations

$$\tau_1 = (\Leftrightarrow \tau_2 - q)/(\tau_2 - \Leftrightarrow) \qquad (17)$$
$$\text{and } f_1 = (\tau_2 - \Leftrightarrow)/(\tau_2 - \tau_1) \qquad (18)$$

The evaluation of τ_2 might be made by studying the additional survival of those members of the cohort who had survived after a time much longer than τ_1.

Conversion of t_i^2 to $t_{i\%}$

For a homogeneous cohort with τ known the set of values of t_i^+ can be converted to a set of values of t_i by use of Equation 8. The mean value of δ_i is τ, but τ is not to be added to each of value of t_i^+: instead a set of values of δ_j is calculated by use of Equation 2 with t given the N values corresponding to the midpoints of the risers on the staircase function S, and these values are assigned to the N values of t_i^+ by a random process. There are N! ways of making this random assignment and there may be some advantage in using more than one (but not taking the average, which would cause all values of δ_i to approach τ).

An extension of this procedure may be used for a heterogeneous cohort.

Analysis of Survival Time of Two Cohorts

As an example we discuss first a cohort of 40 patients with 22 survivors at the termination of the study (Table 4). The values of Σt (374 mo) and Σt^+

(1258 mo) lead by Equation 5 to $<\tau> = 91$ mo. Similarly, the values of Σt^2 and $\Sigma(t^+)^2$ lead by Equation 12 to $<\tau^2>^{1/2} = 109$ mo. A third value is 97 mo, given by the value S = 22/40 at the time $<t^+> = 57.2$ mo, and the mean of the three values of τ is 99 mo.

A second example is that of 61 patients with 29 survivors and with other kinds of cancer (Table 5). A similar analysis leads to $<\tau^+> = 62$ mo, $<\tau^2>^{1/2} = 72$ mo, and $\tau(S) = 68$ mo, mean 67 mo.

Indication of heterogeneity of each of these two cohorts is provided by the analysis of the corresponding subcohorts consisting of those members alive at any time during one year, taken as 1986, leaving 3.5 years during which the additional survival times were observed. These 1986 cohorts would be depleted in the short-lived subcohorts, so that the values of τ would tend toward the values for the long-lived subcohorts. For the 1986 cohort of Table 4, 25 patients with 18 survivors on Jan. 1, 1990, the values $<\tau^+> = 120$ mo, $<\tau^2>^{1/2} = 123$ mo, and $\tau(S) = 124$ mo, mean 122 mo, are found, and for the 1986 cohort of Table 5, 32 patients with 18 survivors, the values are $<\tau^+> = 70$ mo, $<\tau^2>^{1/2} = 72$ mo, and $\tau(S) = 73$ mo, mean 72 mo.

This analysis of the 1986 cohort permits the resolution of each of the cohorts of Table 4 and 5 into two subcohorts, one consisting of the poor responders to the nutrients and the other of the excellent responders.

We assume that the survival times $\tau = 122$ mo and 72 mo for the 1986 patients apply to the longer-living subcohorts of the two cohorts. Comparison of the number of patients in the 1986 cohort and the full cohorts and their mean values of τ indicates that in each case the subcohort with longer survival constitutes about 80% of the cohort. Analysis of the smaller values of τ then leads to the conclusion that the mean survival time of the 20 poor responders is about 10 mo; that is, only about twice that for the patients who did not follow the regimen. There is no statistical correlation of allocation to the two subcohorts and sex, age, or type of cancer.

Discussion

Some questions about the validity of the results presented in this paper have been raised by statisticians and oncologists who have read it or heard it discussed in seminars. We now respond to these questions by providing some additional information.

First, it has not been contended by the critics that the new biostatistical equations based on the Hardin Jones principle contain errors. It was pointed out, especially in the discussion of a presentation of this paper by one of the authors at a seminar in the statistics department of a leading university, that some of the results are not new. The Hardin Jones principle has been discussed briefly in several books and papers during the last thirty years, but never, except by Jones (1957) and Burch (1976), with any significant discussion of its general validity for homogeneous cohorts of cancer patients. It has also been pointed out to us that several methods of handling cohorts with survivors at the end of a study have been developed, usually without any assumption about the nature of the survival curve. These methods are recognized, however, as being less powerful than the method that we have used, which is based on the acceptance of the Hardin Jones principle. We believe that the existing epidemiological evidence provides strong support of this principle, and that it should be used in all biostatistical studies of mortality data for cohorts of cancer patients, in order to increase the accuracy and reliability of the conclusions drawn from the studies.

Dr James Enstrom suggested to us that there might be a contradiction between the Hardin Jones principle and the Gompertz principle. In 1820, 1825 and 1862 Gompertz pointed out that the logarithm of the total death rate and the death rates for some individual diseases are linear functions of the chronological age, usually doubling about every 8 years. No such great dependence on chronological age is seen in our tables. The explanation of this fact is, we suggest that the Gompertz principle applies to cancer morbidity and thus indirectly, by way of the Hardin Jones principle, also to cancer mortality. The study in this paper relates to the time between morbidity and mortality; that is, it is a discussion of the survival times of patients who have developed the disease and have progressed to essentially the same stage, that of untreatability by conventional therapies.

It has been suggested to us that, instead of this retrospective study, we should have carried out a prospective randomized double-blind study of cancer patients, some of whom would receive 12 g of vitamin C each day and also several tablets containing vitamin E and other nutrients, with the controls receiving many tablets or capsules containing corresponding placebos. One of us has for 17 years been urging that such studies be carried out, but with little success. The two Mayo Clinic studies (Creagan et al., 1979; Moertel et al., 1985), usually referred to as having shown vitamin C to have no value in the control of cancer, are so flawed as to be themselves of no value (Pauling and Herman, 1989).

The study reported in this paper was not planned. The clinician member of this team of authors, a psychiatrist, recognized that of the patients with cancer who were registered with him (sent to him by a family physician or oncologist) before 15 April 1988, those who followed his regimen were surviving much longer than those who were not following the regimen. After he had carried out a preliminary analysis of the mortality data, he suggested to the other author that the collaboration be begun that has resulted in this paper.

A principal reason for our decision to publish this analysis is that so little interest has in the past been shown by granting agencies such as the National Cancer Institute and the American Cancer Society and by medical researchers in carrying out studies of the value of vitamin C and other nutrients in the prevention and treatment of cancer, in spite of the impressive results of the work of Cameron and his associates (see below). We are convinced that at the present time the publication of the results of the careful analysis of observations made on all of the members of a group of cancer patients, some of whom followed the orthomolecular regimen whereas others did not, will have value in calling to the attention of both physicians and patients the possibility that this regimen, as an adjunct to appropriate conventional therapy, may have great value.

One critic of an earlier draft of this paper made the statement that it has no value because the clinician author had recruited 101 volunteers for his project from patients in hospitals, with 33 others (used by us in Tables 1 and 2) having refused to enter the study. This complete misunderstanding by the critic necessitates that we present the history of the study in some detail.

First, the critic is completely unfamiliar with the situation in Canada with respect to medical practice between general practitioners and specialists. Abram Hoffer is a specialized psychiatrist, and therefore cannot see any patient whatever until the patient has first been referred to him by a general practitioner. This is the way in which all of the cancer patients listed in the tables were enrolled. For each patient the date of enrollment is given in the tables.

TABLE 4

Values of survival times for 40 female patients with cancer of the breast, ovary, uterus, or cervix who had received ascorbic acid and other vitamins as an adjunct to other therapy (column 7). Column A gives the date when the patient was first seen by A.H. and entered into this study; it is also the date when the administration of vitamin C and the other vitamins was begun. Column B gives the number of months between the diagnosis of cancer and the date in column A. The date of death or the state of health on January 1, 1990 is given in column C. Column AA gives the rate of intake of ascorbic acid in g/d.

		A	Age	Type	B	Treatment[a]	AA	C	t or t[+]
5.	Y.A.	07/86	48	Breast	1	R	10	Well	41 +
10.	M.B.	07/85	46	Breast	1	S,R	1.2	Well	53 +
19.	B.D.	02/83	40	Uterus	24	S,R	6	Well	82 +
20.	J.E.	10/84	49	Breast	18	S,R	12	Died 12/85	14
21.	M.E.	10/86	47	Breast	18	S,C	12	Died 08/88	22
23.	BDo.	05/82	41	Ovary	12	S,R	6	Well	91 +
25.	L.H.	07/81	38	Breast	5	S,C	1.2	Died 06/83	23
27.	J.H.	12/83	46	Breast	4	S,R	10	Well	73 +
29.	K.F.	06/84	48	Ovary	2	S,C	1.2	Died 12/86	30
35.	M.H.	11/82	56	Breast	12	S,C	12	Alive	85 +
36.	D.J.	10/83	70	Breast	24	S,C	6	Died 08/88	58
38.	L.K.	11/84	65	Breast	1	S,R,C	1.2	Alive	61 +
40.	B .K.	10/85	58	Breast	1	S,R	12	Well	50 +
41.	C.L.	08/84	38	Uterus	0	N	12	Well	64 +
44.	M.C.	08/84	69	Breast	2	S,R	1.2	Well	64 +
48.	E.M.	12/86	39	Breast	18	S	1.2	Well	35 +
53.	H.M.	07/81	41	Breast	1	S,C	1.2	Died 04/82	9
55.	V.M.	03/86	56	Breast	42	S	4	Well	45 +
60.	S.S.	03/83	37	Cervix	2	N	9	Well	81 +
61.	M.N.	08/82	65	Breast	12	S,R	1.2	Died 12/85	40
62.	U.T.	06/83	47	Breast	15	S	8	Well	78 +
63.	B.O.	02/85	45	Breast	1	S	12	Well	58 +
67.	M.Pl.	07/86	46	Cervix	72	S,R,C	12	Died 10/86	3
75.	I.S.	12/78	58	Uterus	5	S,C	3	Died 10/79	10
82.	M.W.	03/82	50	Breast	12	R ,C	12	Died 06/86	51
83.	R-S	10/84	52	Breast	23	S,C,R	18	Died 05/88	43
88.	D.K.	10/86	56	Breast	0	S,C	12	Well	38 +
90.	N.S.	06/86	56	Uterus	8	R	12	Died 04/87	10
91.	E.P.	05/80	69	Uterus	0	S,C,R	3		117 +
93.	M.Y.	09/86	71	Breast	1	S,R	12	Well	39 +
108.	W.F.	11/87	43	Breast	6	S,C	12	Died 05/88	6
111.	S.C.	07/87	41	Ovary	8	S	12	Died 11/88	16
116.	A.A.	09/87	68	Ovary	19	S	12	Died 09/88	12

		A	Age	Type	B	Treatment[a]	AA	C	t or t+
117.	G.J.	04/87	46	Breast	36	S,C,R	4	Well	32 +
118.	S.V.	09/87	49	Breast	0	R	12	Well	27 +
120.	A.H.	03/88	73	Cervix	36	R	12	Died 06/88	3
124.	G.C.	03/88	60	Breast	21	S,C	6	Well	21 +
129.	G.S.	11/87	45	Breast	12	S,R	12	Well	25 +
130.	E.W.	07/87	62	Ovary	9	S,C	12	Died 03/88	8
133.	C.W.	12/87	41	Breast	60	S,C	12	Died 03/89	16

[a] S = surgery, R = radiation, C = chemotherapy, N = no treatment

Dr Hoffer had nothing to do with the selection of any of these patients. For the most part, he first saw or heard of them when they first appeared in his office, and he had the patient's file before him. The patients had cancer in an advanced stage, mainly untreatable (with little hope by the physician that any conventional treatment would have more than a palliative effect) but they were ambulatory at the time of registration with him, whereas Cameron's patients were hospitalized at the beginning of their vitamin C regimen (Cameron and Campbell, 1974; Cameron, Campbell and Jack, 1975; Cameron and Pauling, 1974,1976,1978,1979).

The first few patients in this study had been referred to the psychiatrist because of having shown severe depression, and the later ones, who usually suffered from anxiety, because the physicians in the area were beginning to think that the Hoffer regimen, in addition to appropriate conventional therapy, might have significant value for patients with advanced cancer. Dr Hoffer discussed with each patient the nature of the regimen and expressed the hope that their probable future would be improved by this treatment. It was his intention that every patient would follow the same regimen.

There were, however, 33 of the 134 patients who did not follow the regimen. In no case did this occur through action by Dr Hoffer. Some patients were discouraged from following it by the practitioner after Dr Hoffer had sent him his findings and treatment recommendations. Also, some were in the middle of a course of chemotherapy and were so sick with nausea and vomiting that they could not ingest the vitamins, and some of the patients

TABLE 5

Values of survival times for 61 patients with several kinds of cancer who had received ascorbic acid and other vitamins as an adjunct to other therapy (column 8). Column A gives the date when the patient was first seen by A.H. and entered into this study; it is also the date when the administration of vitamin C and the other vitamins was begun. Column B gives the number of months between the diagnosis of cancer and the date in column A. The date of death or the state of health on January 1, 1990 is given in column C. Column AA gives the rate of intake of ascorbic acid in g/d.

		A	Age	Sex	Type	B	Treatment[a]	AA	C	t or t+
1.	E.R.	04/84	64	F	Lung	4	R	12	Well	68+
2.	E.B.	03/86	63	M	Lung	1	N	20	Died 02/87	14
3.	R.B.	07/82	68	M	Mesothelioma	12	R	18	Died 12/82	5
6.	C.B.	01/80	72	M	Sarcoma	24	R	12	Died 08/89	115
11.	R.M.	03/84	25	M	Lymphoma	16	R,C	12	Well	69+
15.	S.B.	04/86	59	M	Colon	5	S	2	Well	44+
17.	R.D.	04/79	60	M	Glioblastoma	8	S	6	Died 07/80	15
18.	B.D.	06/80	63	M	Vocal cord	72	S,R	12	Well	114+
22.	L.E.	08/8 1	16	F	Ewing's sarcoma	22	R,C	12	Well	100+
24.	M.G.	04/83	62	F	Bladder	6	S,R	12	Died 08/88	64
28.	N.H.	09/82	58	M	Pancreas	17	S	10	Died 11/82	2
33.	C.H.	09/80	53	F	Lung	2	S	2	Died 04/81	7
34.	G.I.	11/86	71	M	Prostate	1 2	S	2	Died 05/87	6
37.	C.K.	03/81	54	F	Lung	4	R,C	12	Well	105+
39.	F.K.	06/85	56	M	Lung	24	R,C	12	Died 11/86	17
42.	J. L.	11/84	52	M	Lung	3	R	12	Died 05/85	6
43.	A.L.	11/86	56	M	Prostate	1	R	12	Well	37 +
45.	I.L.	07/80	73	F	Colon	29	S,R	5	Died 05/81	10
46.	L.L.	12/83	63	F	Abdominal	2	S,C	12	Died 02/85	15
49.	D.M.	05/84	39	F	Abdominal	3	S	15	Well	66 +
51.	T.M.	01/83	35	F	Lung	12	C	12	Died 07/83	6
52.	J.M.	05/86	71	M	Leukemia	1	N	40	Died 02/87	9
54.	T.L.	07/81	67	M	Lung	12	R	4	Died 05/82	6
58.	H.M.	11/86	64	F	Pancreas	24	S	2	Well	37 +
64.	R.D.	11/85	40	M	Kidney-lung	12	S	2	Died 03/88	28
66.	M.P.	02/84	14	M	Lymphoma	48	S,C	3	Well	70 +
58.	K.P.	04/86	56	M	Stomach	6	N	12	Died 07/86	3
69.	M.R.	11/86	8	M	Brain	22	S,R,C	6	Died 05/87	6
70.	M.Q.	12/86	47	F	Intestine	19	S	2	Well	36 +
71.	D.R.	03/85	66	M	Jaw	9	S,R	12	Died 09/85	6
72.	D.Ro	10/85	48	M	Brain	60	S,R,C	12	Died 02/88	28
73.	S.R.	06/86	67	M	Prostate	7	S,R	12	Well	42 +
74.	A.Do	06183	36	M	Lymphoma	2	S,C,R	12	Well	78 +

		A	Age	Sex	Type	B	Treat-ment[a]	AA	C	t or t+
77.	H.S.	09/85	50	M	Leukemia	1	N	6	Died 10187	25
80.	J.W.	11/83	54	F	Colon	60	S	24	Died 12/84	13
84.	A.S.	07/78	59	F	Pancreas	2	N	14-40	Well	137 +
85.	B.S.	08/86	61	M	Liver	12	N	7	Died 12/87	16
86.	D.T.	03/81	40	M	Throat	6	R	12	Well	105 +
87.	I.T.	04/82	30	M	Colon	18	S	12	Well	92+
89.	J.G.	02/82	56	F	Lung	9	R,C	12	Died 03/84	25
92.	J.D.	04/84	61	F	Colon	120	S,R	12	Died 09/85	17
94.	S.W.	08183	63	F	Leukemia	0	N	3	Died 12/89	75
95.	M.M.	09/86	59	F	Colon	0	S	12	Well	39 +
96.	W.B.	06/87	58	F	Kidney	6	S,C	12	Died 11/88	17
97.	D.Bo	09/87	54	F	Lung	0	S	2	Well	27 +
98.	K.A.	06/86	61	M	Prostate	12	R	12	Well	42 +
100.	J.Bu.	06/87	62	F	Bronchus	4	R	12	Died 04188	10
101.	J.B.	11/86	56	F	Bowel	5	R	12	Died 03/88	16
104.	F.C.	11/87	63	M	Leukemia	18	C	12	Well	25 +
105.	G.C.	05/87	77	M	Prostate	24	S,R,C	12	Well	31 +
106.	Ge.C	08/87	71	M	Lung	8	N	12	Died 11/88	17
107.	R.G.	O6/87	70	M	Prostate	11	S,C	12	Died 12/87	6
119.	K.A.	08/87	63	M	Pancreas	2	S	12	Died 05/88	9
121.	K.L.	03/88	41	M	Lymphoma	36	C	12	Alive	21 +
122.	F.L.	07/87	64	F	Colon	48	S,R	12	Well	29 +
123.	C.M.	03/88	56	M	Prostate	6	N	12	Died 01/89	10
125.	F.ML	03/87	73	M	Multiple myeloma	2	R,C	12	Well	27 +
126.	L.N.	09/87	42	F	Kidney	6	S,R	12	Well	26 +
128.	E.S.	07/87	79	M	Abdomen	24	S,R	3-6	Died 06/88	11
132.	C.P.	04/87	36	M	Spinal cord	Long	S	12	Well	32 +
134.	J.P.	06/87	69	M	Prostate	36	R	12	Died 12/89	30

[a] S = surgery, R = radiation, C = chemotherapy, N = no treatment

for themselves decided not to follow the regimen. There is no evidence that the controls (Tables 1 and 2) were significantly different from the patients who followed the regimen (Tables 4 and 5). For example, the fractions of controls who had received conventional therapy (surgery, radiation, chemotherapy) before registration was 85% for the 33 controls and also 85% for the 101 other patients, and the mean age at registration was 53.1, 52.8, 51.9 and 55.3 years for the four cohorts of Tables 1, 2, 4 and 5.

Our conclusion is that 80% of the patients who followed the regimen have a probable survival time 21 times that of the controls (Table 4) or 13 times that of the controls (Table 5), or, for all 81 patients, 16 times that of the 31 controls. The mean survival time of the main subgroup of 31 controls, 5.7 mo, is about what is observed for ambulatory patients who have reached or are close to the terminal stage of cancer, with 85% having received potentially curative or palliative conventional therapy. The much longer mean survival time of 81 of the similar patients who followed the regimen, 92 mo, must surely be attributed to this regimen.

These results may be compared with those found in other studies. In 1976 Cameron and Pauling published values of t and t_i^+, starting from the date of untreatability for 198 patients with cancer of the breast, ovary or uterus in Vale of Leven Hospital, Lochlomondside, Scotland, of whom 18 had received continuously 10 g of sodium ascorbate per day, beginning on the date of untreatability, and 180 had not received this vitamin. The value of τ for the latter, equal to $\Sigma\tau/180$ (no t^+), was 2.2 mo, and the corresponding value for the vitamin C cohort (which had some survivors), evaluated by Equations 5 and I2 and the survival fraction, was 13 mo, 6 times as great. For the patients with other kinds of cancer the ratio was also 6 (9 mo vs 1.5 mo). All of the survival times are smaller than those for the present study because the patients in Scotland were at a more advanced stage when they entered the study, that of untreatability and hospitalization, after which no further potentially curative or palliative treatment (except vitamin C) was administered. The larger ratios in the present study might have resulted from several differences, such as the somewhat larger amounts of vitamin C (12 g/d rather than 10 g/d) and the administration also of other vitamins and minerals in large amounts (somewhat variable, usually niacin or niacinamide 1.5 or 3 g/d, pyridoxine 250 mg/d, other B vitamins in variable amounts, vitamin E 800 I U/d, β-carotene 30,000 IU/d, selenium 200 to 500 μg/d, other minerals); the patients were also given advice about the selection of foods.

On the basis of these results and of those reported by Cameron and his collaborators we strongly recommend that patients with cancer follow the regimen described in this paper, as an adjunct to appropriate conventional therapy.

We also join Ewan Cameron (Cameron, 1974) in recommending that physicians consider administering large amounts of sodium ascorbate by intravenous infusion to patients with advanced cancer. Cameron himself gave intravenous ascorbate, usually 10 g/d for about 10 days, as well as oral ascorbate continued indefinitely, to each of his patients, and other physicians have reported the successful use of intravenous ascorbate (Riordan et al., 1990).

– Linus Pauling & Abram Hoffer

Reprinted by permission from *The Journal of Orthomolecular Medicine* 5(3): 143-154, 1990.

References

Burch, P.R.J.: *The Biology of Cancer, A New Approach*. Baltimore, MD: University Park Press, Baltimore, 1976.

Cameron, E. and Pauling, L. "The orthomolecular treatment of cancer. I. The role of ascorbic acid in host resistance." *Chemical-Biological Interactions*, 9:273-283, 1974.

Cameron, E. and Campbell, A. "The orthomolecular treatment of cancer. II. Clinical trial of high-dose ascorbic supplements in advanced human cancer." *Chemical-Biological Interactions*, 9:285-315, 1974.

Cameron, E.; Campbell, A.; and Jack, T. "The orthomolecular treatment of cancer. III. Reticulum cell sarcoma: double complete regression induced by high-dose ascorbic acid therapy." *Chemical-Biological Interactions*, 11:387-393, 1975.

Cameron, E. and Pauling, L. "Ascorbic acid and the glycosaminoglycans: An orthomolecular approach to cancer and other diseases." *Oncology*, 27:181 -192, 1973.

Cameron, E. and Pauling, L. "Supplemental ascorbate in the supportive treatment of cancer: Prolongation of survival times in terminal human cancer." *Proceedings of the National Academy of Sciences USA*, 73:3685-3689, 1976.

Cameron, E. and Pauling, L. "Supplemental ascorbate in the supportive treatment of cancer: Reevaluation of prolongation of survival times in terminal human cancer." *Proceedings of the National Academy of Sciences USA*, 75: 4538-4542, 1978.

Cameron, E. and Pauling, L. "Experimental studies designed to evaluate the management of patients with incurable cancer." *Proceedings of the National Academy of Sciences USA*, 75: 6252, 1978.

Cameron, E. and Pauling, L. *Cancer and Vitamin C*. Palo Alto, CA: Linus Pauling Institute of Science and Medicine, 1979.

Creagan, E.T.; Moertel, C.G.; O'Fallon, J.R.; Schutt, A.J.; O'Connell, M.J.; Rubin, J.; and Frytak, S. "Failure of high-dose vitamin C (ascorbic acid) therapy to benefit patients with advanced cancer: A controlled trial." *New England Journal of Medicine*, 30, 1:687-690, 1979.

Gompertz, B. "A sketch of an analysis and notation applicable to the estimation of the value of life contingencies." *Philosophical Transactions of the Royal Society*, London, 110:214 -294, 1820.

Gompertz, B. "On the nature of the function expressive of the law of human mortality, and on a new mode of determining the value of life contingencies. In a letter to Francis Bally, Esq. F. R.S. etc." *Philosophical Transactions of the Royal Society*, London, 115:513 -585, 1825.

Gompertz, B. "A supplement to the two papers of 1820 and 1825." *Philosophical Transactions of the Royal Society*, London, 152:511-559, 1862.

Hoffer, A.; Osmond, H.; Callbeck, M.J.; and Kahan, I. "Treatment of schizophrenics with nicotinic acid and nicotinamide." *Journal of Clinical and Experimental Psychopathology*, 18:131-149, 1957.

Jones, H.B. "Demographic consideration of the cancer problem." *Transactions of the New York Academy of Sciences*, 18:298-333, 1956.

Moertel, C.G.; Fleming, T.R.; Creagan, E.T.; Rubin, J.; O'Connell, M.J.; and Ames, M.M. "Highdose vitamin C versus placebo in the treatment of patients with advanced cancer who had no prior chemotherapy." *New England Journal of Medicine*, 312:137 -141, 1985.

Pauling, L. "Biostatistical analysis of mortality data for cohorts of cancer patients." *Proceedings of the National Academy of Sciences USA*, 86:3456-3488, 1989.

Pauling, L. and Herman, Z.S. "Criteria for the validity of clinical trials of treatments of cohorts of cancer patients based on the Hardin Jones principle." *Proceedings of the National Academy of Sciences USA*, 86:6835-6837, 1989.

Riordan, H.D.; Jackson, J.A.; and Schulz, M. "Case study: High-dose intravenous vitamin C in the treatment of a patient with adenocarcinoma of the kidney." *Journal of Orthomolecular Medicine*, 5:5-7, 1990.

Appendix 2

The Adrenalin Adrenochrome System and Cancer

The autonomic nervous system controls physiological responses to stress. Its chemical mediators on the sympathetic side are the catecholamines, dopamine, noradrenalin, and adrenalin, particularly the last two. Concerning noradrenalin and adrenalin, Dr Cannon's original description of the flight or fight mechanism is still valid. An emergency or a perceived emergency is a major stimulus to the autonomic nervous system which releases large amounts of adrenalin and noradrenalin. This prepares the body so it can respond best to the emergency. In animals, an inadequate response will lead to either death (the victim) or to no meal (the predator). A rabbit which responds optimally may escape. A coyote which responds optimally may have a meal. Adrenalin alerts the body, increases heart rate and blood pressure, increases the rate of breathing, and diverts blood from viscera to the muscles where it is most needed. It increases sweating to cool the body. It decreases the sensation of pain. This physiological response has been developed over billions of years and is still fully functional even though civilized mankind very seldom has the same need to respond to emergencies the same as do animals in the wild.

Adrenochrome and Cancer

But adrenalin is very toxic because it elevates the blood pressure. The body must remove it as quickly as possible. To do so, it has developed two main pathways for converting it to other substances. One pathway leads to adrenochrome, which does not elevate blood pressure. The other pathway leads to non indolic derivatives. The second pathway is controlled by several enzymes called amine oxidases. Thus a highly reactive compound which elevates pressure is replaced by other compounds that do not have this property.

Adrenochrome (and the other chrome indoles from noradrenalin and from dopamine) have other properties. Adrenochrome is a mitotic poison – i.e., it decreases the rate of cell division. In heart muscle and in leukocytes about 80 percent of the adrenalin is converted into adrenochrome. And adrenochrome is toxic in other ways. It is an hallucinogen. This is fully described in the book I co-authored in 1967 with Dr Humphry Osmond, The Hallucinogens. There we discussed its biochemical, physiological, and psychological properties. It is a highly reactive compound with a short half-life in the body where it is quickly converted into adrenolutin, 3,5,6 tri hydroxy N-methyl indole, which is also hallucinogenic, and to 5,6 dihydroxy N-methyl indole, which is not. On the contrary, this compound, also called leuko adrenochrome (white adrenochrome), has good anti anxiety properties. These substances circulate in the body. The hallucinogenic properties of adrenochrome and adrenolutin led to our adrenochrome hypothesis of schizophrenia – i.e., that this disease came about due to the increased formation of these oxidation products of adrenalin. For the rest of this discussion I will consider its anti mitotic properties and its hallucinogenic properties.

In our 1967 discussion, we wrote, "Adrenochrome markedly inhibits mitotic rate of cells, probably by interfering in the glucolytic cycles. Bullough found that when mice were stressed by overcrowding, the adrenal medulla increased in size 80 percent. At the same time the epidermal mitotic rate fell 60 percent. In vitro adrenaline had no anti mitotic effect on epidermis but when it was injected it did. In contrast, adrenochrome was anti mitotic both in vitro and in vivo. Bullough suggested that during stress the increased quantity of adrenaline was converted into adrenochrome which produced the antimitosis."

These two properties, anti mitosis and hallucinogenic, suggest that it is involved in two conditions: the control of mitosis in the body; and schizophrenia. Elsewhere I have suggested that schizophrenia is a defense mechanism against stress which has gone too far. It is highly likely that since the adrenochrome is present in the body that it would be used to control excess mitosis and that it is involved in the prevention of cancer. This is the hypothesis I will elaborate – i.e., that too little adrenochrome will increase incidence of cancer and decrease the incidence of schizophrenia, while too much will decrease the incidence of cancer and increase the incidence of schizophrenia.

Small amounts of adrenalin are produced all the time even when asleep, but during the day and when exposed to stress the amount is increased. The continual, even if fluctuating, level of adrenalin will ensure a constant production of adrenochrome and its conversion to adrenolutin and other indoles. I suggest that this is one of the mechanisms the body uses to deal with excess mitotis. The leukocytes probably destroy abnormal cells by releasing adrenochrome which has the properties of a free radical and will destroy the cell. It is recognized that pro oxidants are needed to destroy cancer cells. Adrenochrome is probably the best and safest natural pro oxidant in the body. This hypothesis suggests a number of testable sub hypotheses.

1. *A deficiency in the production of adrenochrome* will increase the incidence of cancer and decrease the incidence of schizophrenia. This can arise from (a) inadequate production of adrenalin; (b) a deficiency of enzymes which convert adrenalin to adrenochrome; (c) a deficiency of oxygen; and (d) a deficiency of auto oxidizing systems such as copper or iron.

A deficiency of adrenalin can arise from a deficiency of tyrosine, but this is highly unlikely. It can also arise from extirpation of the adrenal glands, one of the major sources of adrenalin. It could arise from a lack of stimulation of the sympathetic nervous system. Factors such as staying in bed all day would decrease the need for adrenalin to help control blood pressure. An absence of challenges to the body, both psychological and physical, could also produce a deficiency of adrenalin. It could also come about by the use of anti anxiety drugs and tranquilizers which effectively isolate the individual from stress. Infections are stressful and increase the activity of the immune system. The use of tranquilizers since 1950 has effectively removed this spur to the immune system for many people and may be another factor in decreasing adrenalin and therefore adrenochrome production. Helen Coley Nauts made the very sensible suggestion that the loss of repeated episodes of infection by bacteria since the introduction of antibiotics may be a major factor in the rising prevalence of cancer in the highly industrialized world. According to this hypothesis, repeated infections acted as a spur to re-invigorate the immune system continually. According to the adrenochrome hypothesis, it would act as a spur to increase the production of adrenochrome.

2. *Excessive formation of adrenochrome* will decrease the prevalence of cancer and will increase the prevalence of schizophrenia. This can arise

TABLE 1
A Few Characteristics of the Group with Both Cancer and Schizophrenia

Number	Sex	Type	Schiz first	Alive,years
1	F	Breast	Yes	4
2	F	Thyroid	Yes	4
3	F	Breast	Yes	6
4	F	Breast	Yes	2
5	M	Lymphoma	No	12

from the following factors: (a) an overproduction of adrenalin for prolonged periods of time due to excessive stress of various types; and (b) an increase in the production of adrenochrome due to an increase in the conditions which favor this reaction, such as more of the oxidizing enzymes, too little activity of the other enzymes which convert adrenalin to other non indolic substances, an increase in oxygen tension, an increase in oxidizing metals such as copper or iron, and finally too much inhibition of the reaction by any factor which would normally take adrenalin down the non adrenochrome pathway. If cancer did develop in a schizophrenic person, it would probably be less invasive and easier to treat with a better outcome. Patients with cancer would be less likely to become schizophrenic and patients with schizophrenia would be less likely get cancer.

Both of these propositions are true. Since 1977 I have examined and treated over 780 patients with cancer covering almost the entire spectrum of types of cancers and organs involved. Only five were schizophrenic. Three had cancer of the breast, one had a lymphoma, and one cancer of the thyroid. In every case, the response to treatment was excellent. They are all alive, averaging 6 years. The usual stated life time incidence of schizophrenia is said to be 1 percent. I think it is closer to 2 percent. Therefore I would expect that out of this series I would have seen more than these 5. J.D. Kanofsky and associates concluded that schizophrenic patients have a lower incidence of lung cancer compared to the general population, even though they are much heavier smokers. Psychiatric outpatients smoke at almost twice the rate of the general population. He also found that smoking did not lower their ascorbic acid blood levels as much as it does in other people. This, he thought, lowered their risk on exposure to smoking, but according to this adrenochrome hypothesis, it might equally have arisen from the increased concentration of adrenochrome. Kanofsky pointed out on the basis of a literature search that in general schizophrenics have a higher death rate than do the general public. Some studies have shown they have a greater rate for non lung cancer and a lesser or greater rate for all other cancers. The earlier literature had concluded that cancer was rare in schizophrenics who were catatonic and hebephrenic, terms no longer in general use. On the contrary, the death rate from cancer in paranoid schizophrenics was higher than it was in the general population. The only clear finding is the decrease in lung cancer. Perhaps if they were non smokers, their rate of lung cancer would be even lower. I have seen over 4,000 schizophrenic patients since 1952. Currently, I have at least 500 chronic patients under my care. The total incidence of cancer is very low. From my current list only 5 have cancer, the same 5 that I referred to in the cancer series. A few characteristics of this group is shown in Table 1.

Both cancer and schizophrenia are chronic conditions. This data suggests that people destined to get cancer can never make enough adrenochrome to become schizophrenic and do not make enough to control their cancer. The increase in the quantity of oxidants within the environment and the decrease in the amount of antioxidants (vitamin C, vitamin E, etc.) may, therefore, explain why the prevalence of cancer has increased so much over the past two decades. On the other hand, schizophrenics do not make too much adrenochrome all the time. They are, therefore, only partially protected. When they are well, they will make much less and that may not be enough to control the growth of cancer.

The following case histories of schizophrenics with cancer illuminate this hypothesis.

(1) Case # 467, Breast Cancer

Born in 1930, I first saw her in 1977 when she complained she had never been well. She had been treated for schizophrenia with many admissions to hospital and medication as well as electroconvulsive therapy. She had her first attack at age 15. I started her on an orthomolecular program, including niacinamide 3 g, ascorbic acid 3 g, pyridoxine 250 mg, and a sugar free diet. She came back in August 1990. She had remained on the program but had started on niacin instead. She still suffered episodes of depression while on lithium and on the antidepressant prozac. Because of the side effects, she discontinued the prozac. I persuaded her to resume the antidepressant. Later, I started her on anafranil. She became much better. In September 1992 she told me she had been well, had stopped the antidepressant, but when her depression recurred, she went back on. She was still on the vitamin program, including beta carotene 25,000 iu. Then she also told me she had had a lumpectomy in 1986, followed three years later by a mastectomy. She was given tamoxifen, but this had to be stopped as it kept her awake, and she was switched to megace. In January 1993 I changed her antidepressant to zoloft 50 mg. In October 1995 she was well.

(2) Case # 422, Thyroid

Born in 1954, she came to see me about her thyroid cancer in 1992, but I had seen her earlier in July 1977 when she had been admitted to our psychiatric ward. She complained she had been hearing voices for three years. They came on a few months after she had taken LSD on three different occasions. By 1976, when she moved to Victoria, she had been admitted to UBC Health Sciences Center four times and had been diagnosed with schizophrenia. The first admission in Victoria followed a very deep depression with suicide impulses. She suffered many perceptual illusions and hallucinations, was very paranoid and depressed. I started her on an orthomolecular program, which included niacinamide 1.5 g and niacin 1.5 g daily with chlorpromazine 100 mg daily. By the end of 1977 she was well. After that she continued to have a few prolonged episodes of depression and she continued to consume too much alcohol. By mid 1982 she had stopped drinking. In December 1986 she set fire to her apartment as a suicide attempt. Early in 1991 she married and later separated. In May 1992 she was 4.5 months pregnant and she was found to have an enlarged thyroid diagnosed as cancer. Mentally she was normal. In June she had surgery and later was given radioactive iodine for five days. In October 1992 she was well. She had her own business and supervised about 12 workers. Her mood was good. When I saw her for her thyroid cancer, I advised her to take ascorbic acid 6 g, niacinamide 1.5 g, B-complex 50, beta carotene 25,000 iu, selenium 200 mcg, and zinc chelate 30 mg. She had remained on her vitamin B-3 for 10 years after I had first started to treat her for her schizophrenia. On 17 May 1994 she was normal. She was not on the full vitamin program. In May 1996 she was well and employed 30 people.

(3) Case #352, Breast
Born in 1952, I first saw her for cancer on 1 January 1991. This patient was a chronic schizophrenic complicated by alcoholism. I first saw her for these conditions August 1989. She was one of the sickest patients I have seen in many years, having failed to respond to many series of ECT, including outpatient ECT, and to all medication. She was started on a comprehensive orthomolecular program. This combined with dedicated help from a very caring family physician gradually brought her around. By the beginning of 1991 she was very much better, having lost most of her hallucinations and thought disorder. She then discovered a lump in her right breast in January 1991. On 21 March 1991 she had a mastectomy, followed by chemotherapy. She had been on a good orthomolecular program. Her ascorbic acid was then raised to 9 g daily with the addition of beta carotene 25,000 iu, B-complex 50, plus vitamin B-3 around 500 mg daily and the medications needed to control her schizophrenic symptoms. By 30 November 1992 she had almost conquered her drinking problem, was mostly free of schizophrenic symptoms,and there was no recurrence of her cancer. She was careless about following her nutrient program as carefully as she had earlier in the treatment. In July 1996 she was alive.

(4) Case #561, Breast
Born in 1924, she was first seen for cancer on 23 February 1994. I first saw this patient in August 1984, at which time it was considered that she might have Korsakoff's syndrome. However, eventually it turned out that this was not what she had, and in fact she probably had a recurrence of her schizophrenia with depression. She was treated, and I saw her last in May 1987. At that time she was getting along well. When I saw her 23 February 1994, she reported that she was still following the same vitamin program as before plus haldol 2 mg HS to help her sleep. She was mentally normal and had a good relationship with her husband. She then reported that she had had a mastectomy 16 years ago on the right side, with no radiation or following chemotherapy. More recently, she developed a rash under the right arm

which began to weep. She was investigated and it was found she had a slow-growing recurrence of her tumor which was resected, although the surgeon told her he did not get it all. I advised her to take ascorbic acid 4 g t.i.d., niacinamide 500 mg t.i.d., B-complex 50 mg od, selenium 200 mcg od, beta carotene 25,000 iu od, magnesium citrate 50 mg od, enzyme Q_{10} 300 mg per day, and tamoxifen. In July 1996 she was alive.

(5) Case #11, Lymphoma

In December 24, 1982 he complained of acute left upper quadrant pain. His white blood count was 15,000 and he had some fever. He recovered in a few days. On 11 February 1983 he was found to have a huge abdominal mass on the left side. After a few days he left hospital before the investigation was completed but came back a few days later. A few days later he was started on chemotherapy and by 3 March 1983 the mass was smaller and softer. But his oncologist recorded that "he presents with an incurable condition which undoubtedly in the near future will take him away." He was then diagnosed as having paranoid schizophrenia with retroperitoneal lymphoma. On 27 March 1984 I examined him. He was very anxious and worried about his lymphoma. He was then not showing any schizophrenic symptoms and signs. I started him on ascorbic acid 12 g, niacin 1.5 g, B-complex 75s, twice daily, and selenium 150 mcg, all daily. On 4 February 1985 he was admitted to the psychiatric ward. This time he complained of visual illusions, he had a few paranoid delusions and was very depressed. He was admitted again in March 1985 and by then I had rediagnosed him to have schizophrenia, paranoid. He was started on a parenteral slow release tranquilizer because he was not very good at following his medication regime. He was admitted for the last time July 1991 for two days following having taken LSD several times. He had had many admissions over the previous 6 years. For his schizophrenia and to prevent a recurrence of the lymphoma he took niacin between 3 and 12 grams daily, ascorbic acid between 3 and 20 grams daily and any medication he needed, using antidepressants or tranquilizers. The end of 1993 he was free of his lymphoma but his mental condition was unknown. When last seen he was on niacin 6 g and ascorbic acid 20 g, daily. He was alive 31 December 1995 but I had not seen him for several years.

If adrenochrome is synthesized in greater amounts in schizophrenia, there may not be enough adrenochrome to prevent the cancer from appearing but enough to greatly enhance their prognosis. They have all recovered from their cancer. The lymphoma patient is still free of cancer but he is not well mentally. From the much larger series I treated, I cannot recall any cases of cancer. I would expect a much higher incidence of cancer in the schizophrenic group unless there was this incompatibility between the two conditions.

There is other evidence as well. Professor Rudy Falk, University of Toronto Medical School, formerly Chief of Oncology at St. Michael's Hospital, Toronto, estimated that he had seen over 25,000 patients during his long career, and Dr J. Holt, an oncologist in Australia, had seen nearly 18,000 patients over his 41 years of practice. They can not recall a single patient who was also schizophrenic. Dr Holt had been puzzled by this incompatibility for many years. Out of nearly 48,000 cases only five are known to have had schizophrenia. Dr Holt's group also had treated about 700 patients with Ankylosing Spondylitis and he estimated about 6 had been schizophrenic with another 12 disturbed psychiatrically. Apparently, this physical condition did not protect against schizophrenia.

It occurred to me that this protective effect might also be found in the most closely related relatives of these patients – i.e., parents, siblings, and children. These relatives do have some evolutionary advantage. Over the past year I have asked each cancer and each schizophrenic patient I have seen about the presence of either condition in their first order relatives. The results of this clinical survey are shown in Table 2.

Chi Sq. for the distribution for the last two columns is 18 Table 2, i.e., $P<.001$. For the distribution of schizophrenic patients only between the two groups, it is 11.1 and for cancer cases only it is 22.

About 12 percent of the cancer relatives developed cancer. From the schizophrenic relatives only 6 percent did. From the cancer relatives only 2 (0.3 percent) had schizophrenia. The incidence among the general population is between 1 and 2 percent, which from this group should yield between 5 and 10 patients. And from the schizophrenic relatives 12 had cancer. This data supports the hypothesis – i.e., that patients liable to get cancer are much less apt to get schizophrenia and that patients who have or have had schizophrenia are much less apt to have had cancer. Patients

TABLE 2
The Presence of Cancer and Schizophrenia in First Order Relatives of Patients With Cancer or Schizophrenia.

	Number of Relatives			
	Index	Family Members	Schiz	Cancer
Schiz.	83	394	21 (5%)	24 (6%)
Cancer	86	582	2 (.03%)	64 (11%)

with a predisposition to cancer do not make enough adrenochrome to become psychotic, while other people who only make enough adrenochrome now and then will get schizophrenia and will be protected to a degree from getting cancer. And schizophrenic patients who do get cancer will have a much better outlook with treatment. This inverse association between these two killing diseases, cancer which destroys life and schizophrenia which destroys normal life, lead to the prediction that if a patient has cancer and then develops schizophrenia the cancer will be destroyed by the adrenochrome.

My first cancer case in 1960 who was psychotic for at least two months perhaps represents one of these cases. Perhaps his recovery was due to the combination of his psychosis which cleared very rapidly on niacin and ascorbic acid, the vitamins, and the cobalt bomb radiation.

Further suggesting the validity of this hypothesis is a study by J.S. Brown and H.D. Foster examining the geographical relationship between the prevalence of schizophrenia and selenium deficiency in the soil. Their careful detailed examination of 9 surveys led to the conclusion that there is a connection between selenium deficiency and the prevalence of schizophrenia and to the suggestion that selenium supplementation might be valuable in preventing and treating schizophrenic patients. There is also a similar relationship between the prevalence of esophageal cancer and selenium deficiency. This appears to suggest that both schizophrenia and cancer ought to be positively related and they are not. It is possible that a deficiency of selenium increases the probability of developing both diseases, but that it plays a much greater role in preventing cancer. Thus both

FIGURE 1
Effect of Having Pyrroluria on Cancer Survival

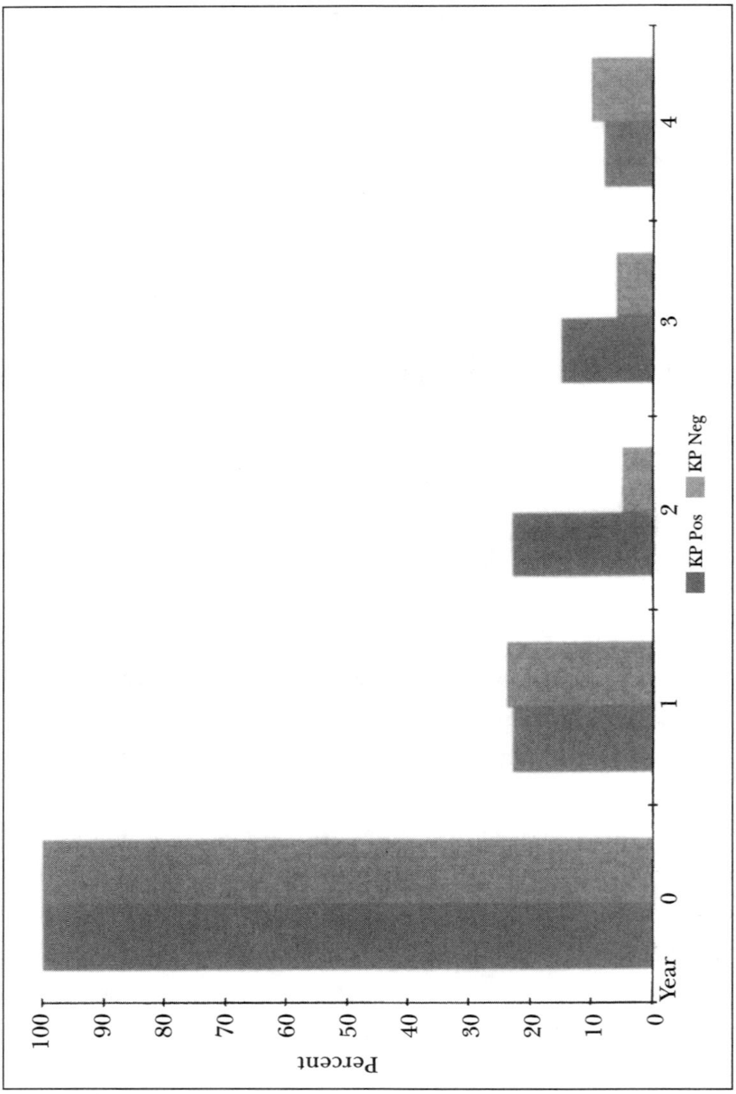

are increased in the absence of enough selenium, but at the same time the association between the two diseases is negative.

Pyrroluria and Cancer

Kryptopyrrole (KP) is found in the urine of the majority of schizophrenic patients and in very few normal people, as we have shown in our studies and Eva Edelman has reviewed comprehensively. It is highly correlated with schizophrenia and its presence established the diagnosis, pyrroluria. It is also present in some patients with cancer, especially if they have cancer of the lung. Seven out of 8 patients with lung cancer were positive for KP, while 4 out of 4 tested after treatment were negative. Two of 7 ovarian and uterine cancer patients were positive. From both groups 80 percent had pyrroluria, but from all other cancers 24 out of 79 or 30 percent were positive. In a previous review of the psychophysiology of cancer, I summarized the cancer literature which showed that lung and ovarian cancers had the highest incidence of psychotic change, usually a form of dementia. This group also had the highest incidence of KP in their urine.

This puzzled me for many years. In thinking about these results, it occurred to me that perhaps the presence of this factor might have an effect on survival. I examined the urine of 34 cancer patients for KP. Only one had been given any vitamin therapy. Thirteen excreted KP and they survived 647 days after their urine was tested. Four lived at least 3 years. The mean survival of the 21 without the factor was 297 days. Three lived at least 3 years. This is shown in Figure 1.

If the adrenochrome hypothesis is valid there will be a correlation between schizophrenia and adrenochrome formation and also between this disease and the presence of KP in the urine. Thus the presence of KP would be a marker for increased adrenochrome formation. Dr O. O'Reilly, a research colleague, also examined urines for KP and he found that cancer patients with KP lived 40 days longer on average than patients who were negative. This was a 10 percent increase in longevity in cancer patients, none of whom were treated with vitamin supplements.

Natural Defense System Against Cancer

To control cancer one needs two sets of reactions. (1) Pro oxidants – e.g., adrenochrome – are used by the body to destroy the tumor cells. Leukocytes kill by discharging free radicals into the bacteria or cell they are attacking. Adrenochrome is a natural superb free radical. (2) Antioxidants neutralize the free radicals as soon as their work is done to prevent injury to other cells and tissues. The adrenalin-adrenochrome system provides a very good system for controlling mitosis. The adrenalin is maintained by repeated exposure to stress. The adrenalin is converted to adrenochrome and is used by the body as needed, and the excess is neutralized by conversion into other indoles which are not as toxic. This is done by the natural antioxidants such as ascorbic acid, vitamin E, the carotenes, and other antioxidants found in food.

Treatment For Cancer Based Upon This Hypothesis

This regimen for treating cancer is based on the need to have adequate amounts of adrenochrome as well as the antioxidants.

1. Increase the Production of Adrenalin

(a) by Psychological Means:

Anger will increase the secretion of adrenalin, but it should be mobilized as an attack on the tumor, and not directed inward toward oneself. Many cancer patients have recognized this and use visualization against the tumor. Anger directed against oneself tends to produce depression. The patient must have a combination of anger against the cancer and hope that it will come under control. Too many oncologists have forgotten the powerful effect of hope and therefore by negative hope increase the death rate of their patients

(b) by Bacterial Infection:

About 100 years ago Dr Coley, a New York surgeon, reviewed the clinical evidence then available which indicated that in some patients a serious infection with staphyloccus or streptococcus led to a cure of the cancer. Later, he developed a vaccine which he used very successfully for many years. Infections increase stress on the body which mobilizes the immune system and creates fever which increases the rate of reactions in the body. The combination must increase the production of adrenalin and therefore also of adrenochrome. Similar vaccines are in use today by several physicians with some success.

(c) by Hyperthermia:

This should also increase the secretion of adrenalin and therefore of adrenochrome.

2. Increase Production of Adrenochrome

(a) by an Increase in Enzyme Activity:

Activating the phenolases which catalyze this reaction will cause an increase in activity of the enzymes which oxidize adrenalin to adrenochrome. Decreasing the activity of amine oxidases by using inhibitors should have this effect by forcing more adrenalin into the adrenochrome pathway. Parnate should be a very good amine oxidase inhibitor used in low doses, under 20 mg daily. At this dose level, it will rarely cause side effects, may improve mood, and should increase the formation of adrenochrome. I have seen psychotic delirious reactions produced by large doses of parnate. The effect on adrenochrome production has not been tested.

(b) by Using Adrenochrome Derivatives.

(c) by Increasing the Amount of Oxygen in the Tissue:

By using oxygen (hyperbaric) or by increasing blood flow through the tumor the amount of oxygen in the tissue can be increased. Tumor tissue tends to be anoxic with the most virulent tumors being the most anoxic. Niacinamide has been shown by J.H. Kim and associates to increase the circulation this way. Niacin would have the same property, perhaps to a larger degree.

(d) by Increasing Auto Oxidation of Adrenalin:

Auto oxidation of adrenalin can be achieved by increasing copper or iron in the body.

The Synergy of Antioxidant Nutrients

Based upon this adrenochrome hypothesis, therapy for cancer should include substances which counteract the hallucinogenic effect of adrenochrome and compounds which facilitate its conversion to other less toxic compounds. Vitamin B-3 (niacin and nicotinamide) is the best antidote to the hallucinogenic properties of adrenochrome and adrenolutin, as it is against d-lysergic acid diethyl amide. The antioxidants will promote the conversion of adrenochrome to leuko adrenochrome and to adrenolutin. These include ascorbic acid, the best water soluble antioxidant, and vitamin E, the best fat soluble antioxidant in the body. It will also include the carotenes, coenzyme Q_{10}, glutathione, the bioflavonoids, and the antioxidant trace element selenium.

Both vitamin C and vitamin B-3 have an enormous range of therapeutic activities. This suggests that except for the two diseases cancer and schizophrenia, which have a direct relationship to adrenochrome, these vitamins have a general systemic effect which reduces the pathological reaction of the body to stress and thus allows the natural repair processes of the body to operate at a more efficient level. Since every disease results from or creates stress on the body because of the impact of increased production of adrenalin and adrenochrome, these anti stress vitamins should have a general therapeutic effect on every disease. Every disease, or every stress related activity, will benefit from the addition of optimum amounts of the B-vitamins, especially B-3, and the other antioxidant nutrients. There is already ample evidence in addition to the evidence presented here that life is extended and its quality enhanced by this program. Niacin prolongs life, vitamin E should do so as it decreases the frequency of coronary disease, and vitamin C prolongs the life of cancer patients. They each work when used alone, but there is a growing consensus that the combination of these antioxidants has a synergistic effect.

For example, K.N. Prasad and associates, using cell cultures, found that using individual vitamins might be effective, ineffective, or even counter productive, depending upon the vitamin, dose, and type of tumor. In contrast the mixture of four vitamins (vitamin C, alpha tocopherol succinate, beta carotene, and retinoic acid) consistently reduced growth of both cell lines studied and enhanced the growth inhibitory effects of chemo-therapeutic agents on these cells. Unprocessed food does not contain only one vitamin. It contains them all even if in very small amounts. It is not surprising that they work better in combination with each other, for that is what nature has been doing since life originated.

Parkinson's disease is another example of a condition which is related to excessive oxidation (autooxidation), yielding too many free radicals. As P. Jenner has observed, "There has been reluctance by scientists, grant-giving bodies, and the pharmaceutical industry to accept that free-radical mechanisms are an important component of neurodegenerative disease. A decade ago the concept was thought facile, but at least now some acceptance has been gained. Nobody is claiming that free radicals explain every unique feature of neurodegenerative disease. Rather, we are proposing that they are a common feature of the process of cell death in most, if not all, such illnesses. If so, the therapeutic rewards may be great. It may become possible to stop or slow the progression of common disorders, such as Alzheimer's or Parkinson's disease, with a single therapeutic approach." I have evidence that the combination of niacin (and perhaps niacinamide as well) and antioxidants will be therapeutic for Parkinson's disease. Over the past 30 years I have treated patients with Parkinson's disease with niacin, 500 mg t.i.d. to 1000 mg t.i.d. It has been very effective in removing psychiatric symptoms, but has been of no value in treating the neurological component. This disease is considered to be a dopamine deficiency disease and is treated with large doses of l-dopa, in one form or another. But large doses produce schizophrenic-like symptoms, the higher the dose the greater the incidence.

This is not surprising since dopachrome must have properties similar to adrenochrome – i.e., it is an hallucinogen. More likely Parkinson's disease is a combination of too little dopamine and too much dopachrome – i.e., there is excessive conversion of dopamine into dopachrome. Dopachrome is neurotoxic, and increasing destruction of neurons will accelerate the development of the disease while at the same time masking some of the symptoms. Adrenalin is oxidized to oxidized adrenalin losing one electron. In the presence of the NAD $\leftrightarrow$ NADH system the oxidized adrenalin is reduced back to adrenalin and the cycle continues. When there is too little NAD or NADH or both, another electron is lost and adrenochrome is formed. This last reaction is irreversible. Vitamin B-3, therefore, can decrease the production of adrenochrome. This has not been tested experimentally, but in a recent series of reports Professor J.G D. Birkmayer and his associates at the Birkmayer Institute for Parkinson Therapy, in Vienna, Austria, studied a stable form of NADH. They found that their stable preparation using 5 mg doses was therapeutic for Parkinson's disease, for Alzheimer's, and for depression. As they concluded, "When we first used NADH with regard to its clinical efficacy the effect was not convincing. This was most likely due to the rapid dissolution (approximately 10-15 minutes) of the capsule leading to a released of NADH into the acid conditions of the stomach. Since NADH is rapidly oxidized below pH 7.6 the conditions in the stomach will inactivate NADH by converting it to NAD. The investigations of this report were therefore performed with NADH capsules coated with an acid stable film and a release time of 2-3 hours. With this galenic formulation of NADH an improvement in disability could be achieved which was comparable to that of intravenously applied NADH."

The lipid soluble vitamin E also has some therapeutic value in treating Parkinson's disease. Coenzyme Q_{10} is coming into prominent use as a powerful antioxidant. A.H.V. Schapira and associates reported that NADH-ubiquinone (Q_{10}) reductase (Complex 1) and NADH cytochrome c reductase activities were reduced in Parkinson's disease in the substantia nigra. It occurred to me that providing both increased amounts of niacin, the precursor or NAD and NADH, and large amounts of coenzyme Q_{10} would be of value in treating cases of Parkinson's disease. I have given this combination to one patient with classical Parkinson's disease. The first one, age 84, had been on the orthomolecular regimen for at least 25 years and he was mentally normal. His program included niacin 1 gram t.i.d. and the usual antioxidants such as ascorbic acid, vitamin E, and selenium. A couple of years ago Parkinson's disease was diagnosed. It was evident in his gait, leg muscle weakness, and tremor. Last year his neurologist started him on sinemet which may have helped slightly but he continued to deteriorate. Late last summer I advised him to add coenzyme Q_{10}, 600 mg daily to his program. Within two weeks he was much better. When I saw him early in July this year, he had regained the use of his limbs, had very little tremor, and was able once more to play golf as had been his habit before. He is on Q_{10} 300 mg daily. His neurologist was very surprised at the marked improvement.

Another patient had difficulty walking for many years. Her walk closely resembled the walk of a patient with Parkinson's disease, and the diagnosis had been considered by her physician. I tried to help her for several years with no relief. But after she was started on Q_{10} 300 mg daily, within one month there was a marked improvement in her walk and also in her mood.

With a combination of vitamin B-3 plus antioxidants, especially Q_{10}, it may be possible to prevent and to treat Parkinson's disease. The treatment would have to be started as early as possible before too may neurons have been destroyed by the adrenochrome or dopachrome. The niacin will protect against the psychological side effects of the l-dopa treatment and the antioxidants will protect against the neuromuscular effects of the disease. One could then use l-dopa without the patient having to suffer its toxic consequences and their lives would be prolonged.

Works Cited

Agnew, N. and Hoffer, A. "Nicotinic Acid Modified Lysergic Acid Diethylamide Psychosis." *Journal of Mental Science,* 101 (1955): 12-27.

Altschul, R.; Hoffer, A.; and Stephen, J.D. "Influence of Nicotinic Acid on Serum Cholesterol in Man." *Archives of Biochemistry and Biophysics,* 54 (1955): 558-559.

Anonymous. "Vitamin Supplements are Seen as No Guard Against Diseases" and "Study Sees No Benefit in Vitamins on Cancer or Heart Disease.' *New York Times,* April 14, 1994.

Beahrs, O.H.; Henson, D.E.; Hutter, R.V. et al (eds). *Manual for Staging of Cancer, 4th ed.* Philadelphia, PA: Lippincott, 1992.

Bedrick, A.E.; Ramasamy, G.; and Tchertkoff, V. "Histochemical determinations of copper, zinc and iron in pigmented nevi and melanoma." *American Journal of Dermatopathology,* 13 (1991), 575-578.

Benade, L.; Howard, T.; and Burke, D. "Synergistic killings of Ehrlich ascites carcinoma cells by ascorbate and 3 amino-1,2, 4-triazole." *Oncology,* 23 (1969): 33-43.

Benton, D. and Cook, R. "The impact of selenium supplementation on mood." *Biological Psychiatry,* 29 (1991): 1092-1098.

Bindoli, A.; Rigobello, M.P.; and Deeble, D.J. "Biochemical and toxicological properties of the oxidation products of catecholamines." *Free Radical Biology and Medicine,* 13 (1992): 391 - 405.

Birkmayer, J.G.D. *Nicotinamide adenine dinucleotide (NADH): The new therapeutic approach for improving dementia of the Alzheimer's type.* Vienna, Austria: Forschungs - und Lehreinrichtung des Birkmayer Instituts fur Parkinsontherapie. (Available from Menuco Corp., 350 Fifth Ave., Suite 7509, New York, NY 10118.)

Birkmayer, J.G.D. and Birkmayer, W. "The coenzyme nicotinamide adenine dinucleotide (NADH) as biological antidepressive agent." [Experience with 205 patients.] *New Trends in Clinical Neuropharmacology,* 5 (1991): 19-25.

Birkmayer, J.G.D.; Vrecko, C.; Volc, D.; and Birkmayer, W. "Nicotinamide adenine dinucleotide (NADH) — a new therapeutic approach to Parkinson's disease." *Acta Neurologica Scandanvica,* 87, Supp 146 (1993): 32-35.

Birkmayer, W. and Birkmayer, J.G.D. "Nicotinamide adenine dinucleotide (NADH): The new approach in the therapy of Parkinson's disease." *Annals of Clinical and Laboratory Science* 19 (1989): 38-43.

Brock, K.E.; Berry, G.; Mock, P.A.; Maclennan, R.; Truswell, A.S.; and Brinton, L.A. "Nutrients in diet and plasma and risk of in situ cervical cancer." *Journal of the National Cancer Institute,* 80 (1988): 580-585.

Brown, J.S. and Foster, H.D. "Schizophrenia: An update of the selenium deficiency hypothesis." *Journal of Orthomolecular Medicine,* 1996.

Burke, K.E. "Oral and topical L-selenomethionine protection from ultraviolet-induced sunburn, tanning and skin cancer." *Journal of Orthomolecular Medicine,* 1992.

Burke, K.E.; Combs, G.F. Jr.; Gross, E.G.; Bhuyan, K.C. and Abu-Libdeh, H. "The effects of topical and oral L-selenomethionine on pigmentation and skin cancer induced by ultraviolet irradiation." *Nutrition and Cancer,* 17 (1992): 123-37.

Cameron, E. and Pauling, L. *Cancer and Vitamin C*. Palo Alto, CA: Linus Pauling Institute of Science and Medicine, 1979; New York , NY: W.W. Norton and Co., 1979; revised edition, Philadelphia, PA: Camino, 1993.

Cameron, E. and Campbell, A. "The orthomolecular treatment of cancer II. Clinical trial of high-dose ascorbic supplements in advanced human cancer." *Chemical-Biological Interactions*, 9 (1974): 285-315.

Cameron, E. "Protocol for the use of vitamin C in the treatment of cancer." *Medical Hypothesis*, 36 (1991): 190-194.

Cameron, E. and Campbell, A. "Innovation vs quality control: An unpublishable, clinical trial of supplemental ascorbate in incurable cancer." *Medical Hypothesis*, 36 (1991): 185-189.

Campbell, A.; Jack, T and Cameron, E. "Reticulum cell sarcoma: Two complete 'spontaneous' regressions, in response to high-dose ascorbic acid therapy. A report on subsequent progress." *Oncology*, 48 (1991): 495-497.

Canner, P.L.; Berge, K.G.; Wenger, N.K.; Stamler, J.; Friedman, L.; Prineas, R.J.; and Freidewald, W. "Fifteen year mortality in coronary drug project; Patients long term benefit with niacin." *American College of Cardiology*, 8 (1986): 1245-1255.

Cetinkaya, N. and Cetinkaya, D. "Serum copper, zinc levels and copper zinc ratio in healthy women and women with gynecological tumors." *Biological Trace Element Research*, 18 (1988): 29-38.

Challem, J. *The Nutrition Reporter*, 8: January, 1997.

Chaplin, D.J.; Horsman, M.P.; and Aoki, D.S. "Nicotinamide, Fluosol DA and Carbogen: A strategy to reoxygenate acutely and chronically hypoxic cells in vivo." *British Journal of Cancer*, 63 (1990): 109-113.

Chaplin, D.J.; Peters, C.E.; Horsman, M.R. and Trotter, M.J. "Drug induced perturbations in tumor blood flow: Therapeutic potential and possible limitations." *Radiotherapy and Oncology*, 20, Supp 1 (1991): 93-101.

Chen, C.A.; Hwang, J.L.; Kuo,C.Y.; Hsieh, C.Y.; and Huang, S.C. "Serum copper and zinc levels in patients with cervical cancer." *Journal of the Formosan Medical Association*, 8 (1990): 677-682.

Chen, G. and Pan, Q.C. "Potentiation of the antitumor activity of cisplatin in mice by 3-aminobenzamide and nicotinamide." *Cancer, Chemotherapy and Pharmacology*, 22 (1988): 303-307.

Cheraskin, E. *The Vitamin C Controversy: Questions and Answers*. Wichita, KS: Bio-Communications Press, 1988.

Cheraskin, E.; Rinsgdorf, W.M. and Brecher, A. *Psychodietetics*. New York, NY: Stein and Day, 1974.

Clancy, J.; Hoffer, A.; Lucy J.; Osmond H.; Smythies J.; and Stefaniak B. "Design and planning in psychiatric research as illustrated by the Weyburn Chronic Nucleotide Project." *Bull Men Clinic*, 18 (1954): 147-153.

Comstock, G.W.; Helzlsouer, K.H.; and Bush, T.L. "Prediagnostic serum levels of carotenoids and vitamin E as related to subsequent cancer in Washington County, Maryland." *American Journal of Clinical Nutrition*, 53 (1991): 260S-264S.

Corman, L.C. and Davidson , R.A. "Why clinical trials fail: The hidden assumptions of clinical trials." *Southern Medical Journal*, 85 (1992): 117-118.

Cousins, N. *Anatomy of an Illness*. New York, NY: W.W. Norton & Co., 1979.

de Vries, N. and Snow, G.B. "Relationship of vitamins A and E and beta-carotene serum levels to head and neck cancer patients with and without second primary tumors." *European Archives Oto-rhino-laryngology*, 247 (1990): 368-370.

Dhalla, K.S.; Ganguly, P.K.; Rupp, H.; Beamish, R.E.; and Dhalla, N.S. "Measurement of adrenolutin as an oxidation product of catecholamines in plasma." *Molecular and Cellular Biochemistry*, 87 (1989): 85-92.

Diez, M.; Cerdan, F.J.; Arroyo, M.; and Baiibrea, J.L. "Use of the copper/zinc ratio in the diagnosis of lung cancer." *Cancer*, 63 (1989): 726-730.

Ebadi, M. and Swanson, S. "The status of zinc, copper and metallothionein in cancer patients." *Progress in Clinical and Biological Research*, 259 (1988): 161-175.

Edelman, E. *Natural Healing for Schizophrenia: A Compendium of Nutritional Methods*. Eugene, OR: Borage Books, 1996.

Fahn, S. and Cohen, G. "The oxidant stress hypothesis in Parkinson's disease: Evidence supporting it." *Annals of Neurology*, 32 (1992): 804-812.

Falk, R. Personal communication, 1995.

Fornstedt, B. "Role of cetechol autooxidization in the degeneration of dopamine neurons." *Acta Neurologica Scandanvica*, Supp 129 (1990): 12-14.

Foster, H.F. *Health, Disease and The Environment*. Boca Raton, FL: CRC Press, 1992.

Frei, B.; England, L.; and Ames, B.N. "Ascorbate is an outstanding antioxidant in human blood plasma." *Proceedings of the Natural Academy of Sciences*, 86 (1989): 6377-6381.

Gal, D.; Lischinsky, S.; Friedman, M.; and Zinder, O. "Prediction of the presence of ovarian cancer at surgery by an immunochemical panel: CA 125 and copper-to-zinc ratio." *Gynecologic Oncology*, 35 (1989): 246-250.

Gerson, M. "Dietary considerations in malignant neoplastic disease. A preliminary report." *The Review of Gastroenterology*, 12 (1945): 419-425.

Gerson, M. "Effects of a combined dietary regime on patients with malignant tumors." *Experimental Medicine and Surgery*, 7 (1949): 299-317.

Goode, H.F.; Kelleher, J.; Walker, B.E.; Hall, R.I.; and Guillou, P.I. "Cellular and muscle zinc in surgical patients with and without gastrointestinal cancer." *Clinical Science*, 79 (1990): 247-252.

Gopalakrishna, R. "Vitamin E succinate inhibits protein kinase C; correlation with its unique inhibitory effects on cell growth and transformation." *Second Denver Conference on Nutrition and Cancer*, Sept 7-11, 1994, Denver, CO.

Goth, A. and Litmann, I. "Ascorbic acid content in human cancer tissue." *Cancer Research*, 8 (1948): 349-351.

Gotoh, H.; Nomura, T.; Nakajima, C.; Hasegawa, C.; and Sakamoto, Y. "Inhibiting effects of nicotinamide on urethane-induced malformations and tumors in mice." *Mutation Research*, 199 (1988): 55-63.

Gupta, S.K.; Shukla, V.K.; Vaidya, M.P.; Roy, S.K.I.; and Gupta, S. "Serum trace elements and Cu/zn ratio in breast cancer patients." *Journal of Surgical Oncology*, 46: 178-181.

Hager,T. *Force of Nature: The Life of Linus Pauling*. New York, NY: Simon and Schuster, 1995.

Hanck, A.B. "Vitamin C and cancer." *Nutrition, Growth and Cancer*. New York, NY: Alan R. Liss., Inc., 1988.

Hawkins, D.R. and Pauling, L., eds. *Orthomolecular Psychiatry*. San Francisco, CA: W.H. Freeman and Co., 1973.

Heinonen, O.P. and The Alpha-Tocopherol, Beta Carotene Cancer Prevention Study Group. "The Effect of Vitamin E and Beta Carotene on the Incidence of Lung Cancer and Other Cancers in Male Smokers." *New England Journal of Medicine*, 330 (1994): 1029-1035.

Hisake, T.; Furumoto, K.; Nozaka, K.; Kono, K.; Odachi ,T.; Mizumoto, K.; Nischimura, D.; and Koga, S. "Serum zinc and copper changes after gastrectomy in aged patients with gastric cancer." *Japanese Journal of Surgery*, 18 (1988): 158-163.

Hoffer, A.; Osmond, H.; and Smythies, J. "Schizophrenia: A New Approach. II. Results of a Year 's Research." *Journal of Mental Science*, 100 (1954): 29-45.

Hoffer, A. "Adrenochrome and adrenolutin and their relationship to mental disease." *Psychotropic Drugs*. (Garattini, S. and Ghetti, V., eds.): 10-20. London, UK: Elsevier Press, 1957.

Hoffer, A.; Osmond, H.; Callbeck, M.I.; and Kahan, I. "Treatment of Schizophrenia with Nicotinic Acid and Nicotinamide." *Journal of Clinical Experimental Psychopathology*, 18 (1957): 131-158.

Hoffer, A. and Osmond, H. "Double blind clinical trials." *Journal of Neuropathology*, 2 (1961): 221-227.

Hoffer, A. "The effect of adrenochrome and adrenolutin on the behavior of animals and the psychology of man." *International Review of Neurobiology*, 4 (1962): 307-371.

Hoffer, A. and Osmond, H. "Some problems of stochastic psychiatry." *Journal of Neuropsychiatry*, 5 (1963): 97-111.

Hoffer, A. "Faith, hope and chemotherapy." *Chemotherapy*, 9 (1964): 263-274.

Hoffer, A. "Treatment of organic psychosis with nicotinic acid (a single case)." *Disorders of the Nervous System*, 26 (1965): 358-360.

Hoffer, A. "Treatment of schizophrenia with a therapeutic program based upon nicotinic acid as the main variable." *Molecular basis of some aspects of mental activity, Vol II*. (O. Walaas, ed.). New York, NY: Academic Press, 1967.

Hoffer, A. and Osmond, H. *The Hallucinogens*. New York, NY: Academic Press, 1967.

Hoffer, A. "Five California Schizophrenics." *Journal of Schizophrenia*, 1 (1967): 209-220.

Hoffer, A. "A theoretical examination of double-blind design." *Canadian Medical Association Journal*, 97 (1967): 123-127.

Hoffer, A. "Symposium on statistical aspects of protocol design." Discussion. *Cancer Clinical Investigation Review Committee*, San Juan, Puerto Rico, Dec. 9-10, 1970: 224-229.

Hoffer, A. "The Psychophysiology of Cancer." *Journal of Asthma Research*, 8 (1970): 61-76.

Hoffer, A. "L-Dopa: An Hallucinogen." *Schizophrenia*, 2 (1970): 37 only; and 2 (1970): 127 only.

Hoffer, A. "Mechanism of Action of Nicotinic Acid and Nicotinamide in the Treatment of Schizophrenia." *Orthomolecular Psychiatry*. David Hawkins & Linus Pauling, eds. San Francisco, CA: W.H. Freeman & Co., 1973.

Hoffer, A. "An examination of the double-blind method as it has been applied to megavitamin therapy." *Orthomolecular Psychiatry*, 2 (1973): 107-114.

Hoffer, A. and Osmond, H. "In Reply to The American Psychiatric Association Task Force Report on Megavitamin and Orthomolecular Therapy in Psychiatry." Regina, SK: Canadian Schizophrenia Foundation, 1976.

Hoffer, A. "Some theoretical principles basic to orthomolecular psychiatric treatment." *Ecologic-Biochemical Approaches to Treatment of Delinquents and Criminals*. L.J. Hippchen, ed. New York, NY: Van Nostrand-Reinhold Co., 1978: 31-55.

Hoffer, A. and Walker, M. *Orthomolecular Nutrition: New Lifestyle For Super Good Health*. New Canaan, CT: Keats Publishing Inc., 1978.

Hoffer, A. "The adrenochrome hypothesis of schizophrenia revisited." *Journal of Orthomolecular Psychiatry*, 10 (1981): 98-118.

Hoffer, A. "Oxidation-reduction in the brain." *Journal of Orthomolecular Psychiatry*, 12 (1983): 292-301.

Hoffer, A. *Vitamin B-3 (Niacin)*. New Canaan, CT: Keats Publishing, Inc., 1984.

Hoffer, A. "Dopamine, noradrenalin and adrenalin metabolism to methylated or chrome indole derivatives: Two pathways or one?" *Journal of Orthomolecular Psychiatry*, 14 (1985): 262-272.

Hoffer, A. *Orthomolecular Medicine for Physicians*. New Canaan, CT: Keats Publishing, Inc., 1989.

Hoffer, A. and Osmond, H. "The adrenochrome hypothesis and psychiatry." *Journal of Orthomolecular Medicine*, 5 (1990): 32-45.

Hoffer, A. and Osmond, H. *How To Live With Schizophrenia*. New York, NY: University Books, 1966; new and revised ed., New York, NY: Citadel Press, 1992; millennium ed.,Kingston, ON: Quarry Health Books, 2000.

Hoffer, A. and Pauling, L. "Hardin Jones biostatistical analysis of mortality data for cohorts of cancer patients with a large fraction surviving at the termination of the study and a comparison of survival times of cancer patients receiving large regular oral doses of vitamin C and other nutrients with similar patients not receiving those doses." *Journal of Orthomolecular Medicine*, 5 (1990): 143-154; reprinted in E. Cameron and L. Paulking, *Cancer and Vitamin C*.

Hoffer, A. and Pauling, L. "Hardin Jones biostatistical analysis of mortality data for a second set of cohorts of cancer patients with a large fraction surviving at the termination of the study and a comparison of survival times of cancer patients receiving large regular oral doses of vitamin C and other nutrients with similar patients not receiving these doses." *Journal of Orthomolecular Medicine*, 8 (1993): 1547-167.

Hoffer, A. and Walker, M. *Smart Nutrients — A Guide To Nutrients That Can Prevent and Reverse Senility*. Garden City Park, NY: Avery Publishing Group, 1994.

Hoffer, A. "Chronic schizophrenic patients treated ten years or more." *Journal of Orthomolecular Medicine*, 9 (1994): 737.

Hoffer, A. "Orthomolecular Oncology." *Adjuvent Nutrition in Cancer Treatment*. P. Quillin and R. Michael Williams, eds. Arlington Heights, IL: Cancer Treatment Research Foundation, 1994.

Hoffer, A. "Orthomolecular Oncology and Survival." *Adjuvent Nutrition in Cancer Treatment Symposium*. San Diego, CA, Mar 17-19, 1994.

Hoffer, A. and Walker, M. *Putting It All Together — The New Orthomolecular Nutrition*. New Canaan, CT: Keats Publishing Inc., 1994.

Hoffer, A. *Hoffer's Laws of Natural Nutrition*. Kingston, ON: Quarry Press, 1996.

Hoffer, A. "Schizophrenia: An Evolutionary Defense Against Severe Stress." *Townsend Letter for Doctors and Patients*, 151/152, Feb/March 1996.

Hoffer, A. *Vitamin B-3 and Schizophrenia: Discovery, Recovery, Controversy*. Kingston, ON: Quarry Press, 1997.

Hoffer, J. "Nutrients as biologic response modifiers." *Adjuvent Nutrition in Cancer Treatment* (P. Quillin and R.M. Williams, eds.). Arllington Heights, Il: 1992 Symposium Proceedings, Cancer Treatment Research Foundation and American College of Nutrition, 1993.

Holt, J.A.G. "Letter," September 21, 1993, Perth, Australia: Microwave Therapy Center, 311 Outram St., W. Perth, Australia, 6005.

Horsman, M.R.; Chaplin, D.J.; and Brown, J.M. "Radiosensitization by nicotinamide in vivo: A greater enhancement of tumor damage compared to that of normal tissue." *Radiation Research*, 109 (1987): 479-489.

Horsman, M.R.; Brown, J.M.; Hirst, V.K.; Lemmon, M.J.; Wood, P.J.; Dunphy, E.P.; and Overgaard, J. "Mechanism of action of the selective tumor radiosensitizer nicotinamide." *International Journal of Radiation Oncology Biophysics*, 15 (1988): 685-690.

Horsman, M.R.; Chaplin, D.J.; and Brown, J.M. "Tumor radiosensitization by nicotinamide: A result of improved perfusion and oxygenation." *Radiation Research*, 118 (1989): 139-150.

Horsman, M.R.; Overgaard, J.; Christensen K.L.; Trotter, M.J.; and Chaplin, D.J. "Mechanism for the reduction of tumor hypoxia by nicotinamide and the clinical relevance for radiotherapy." *Biomedica Biochimica Acta*, 48, Supp 251-254 (1989): 2-3.

Horsman, M.R.; Chaplin, D.J.; and Overgaard, J. "Combination of nicotinamide and hyperthermia to eliminate radioresistant chronically and acutely hypoxic tumor cells." *Cancer Research*, 50 (1990): 7430-7436.

Horsman, M.R. and Aoki, D.S. "Nicotinamide, Fluosol DA and Carbogen: A strategy to reoxygenate acutely and chronically hypoxic cells in vivo." *British Journal of Cancer*, 63 (1991): 109-113.

Horsman, M.R.; Kristjansen, P.E.; Mizuno, M.; Christensen, K.L.; Chaplin, D.J.; Quistorff, B.; and Overgaard, J. "Biochemical and physiological changes induced by nicotinamide in a C3H mouse mammary carcinoma and CDF1 mice." *International Journal of Radiation Oncology, Biology, Physics*, 22 (1992): 451-454.

Hostetler, D. "Jacobsons put broad strokes in the niacin/cancer picture." *The D.O.*, 28 (1987): 103-104.

Huxley, J.; Mayr, E.; Osmond, H.; and Hoffer, A. "Schizophrenia as a genetic morphism." *Nature*, 204 (1964): 220-221.

Jacobson, M. and Jacobson, E. "Niacin, nutrition, ADP ribosylation and cancer." *The 8th International Symposium on ADP-Ribosylation*. Fort Worth, TX: Texas College of Osteopathic Medicine, 1987.

Jenner, P. "Oxidative damage in neurodegenerative disease." *The Lancet*, 344 (1994): 796-798.

Jonsson, G.G.; Kjellen, E.; Pero, R.W.; and Cameron, R. "Radiosensitization effects of nicotinamide on malignant and normal mouse tissue." *Cancer Research*, 45 (1985): 3609-3614.

Kallistratos, G.I.; Fasske, E.E.; Karkabouas, S.; and Charal-Ambopoulos, K. "Prolongation of the survival time of tumor bearing wistar rats through a simultaneous oral administration of vitamins C and E and selenium with glutathione." In *Nutrition, Growth & Cancer*. New York, NY: Alan R. Liss, Inc, , 1988: 377-389

Kanofsky, J.D.; Norkus, E.P.; Geller, B.; Lowinger, R.; Kanofsky, P.B. and Kennedy, G.K. "Schizophrenia, lung cancer and vitamin C." Philadelphia, PA: American Psychiatric Association, Poster Session, May 1994.

Kiene, H. "A critique of the double-blind clinical trial." *Alternative Therapies*, 2 (1996): 53-59 & 61-66.

Kim, J.H.; Kim, S.H.; He, S.; Dragovic, J.; and Brown, S. "Use of vitamins as adjunct to conventional cancer therapy." *Second Denver Conference on Nutrition and Cancer*, Denver, CO, Sept 7-11, 1994. *Nutrients in Cancer Prevention and Treatment* (Prasad, K.N.; Santamaria, L. and Williams, R.M., eds.). New Jersey: Humana Press, 1995: 363-72.

Kjellen, E.; Pero, R.W.; Cameron, R. and Ranstam, J. "Radiosensitizing effects of nicotinamide on a C3H mouse mammary adenocarcinoma." *Acta Radiologica Oncology*, 25 (1986): 281-284.

Kjellen, E.; Joiner, M.C.; Collier, J.M.; Johns, H. and Rojas, A. "A therapeutic benefit from combining normobaric carbogen or oxygen with nicotinamide in fractionated x-ray treatments." *Radiotherapy and Oncology*, 22 (1991): 81-91.

Kline, K. "Vitamin E succinate: Mechanisms of action as tumor cell growth inhibitor." Denver, CO: Second Denver Conference on Nutrition and Cancer, Sept 7-11, 1994.

Knekt, P. "Role of vitamin E in the prophylaxis of cancer." *Annals of Medicine*, 23 (1991): 3-12.

Knekt, P.; Aromaa, A.; Maatela, J.; Aaran, R.K.; Nikkara, T.; Hakama, M.; Hakulinen, T.; Peto, R.; and Teppo, L. "Vitamin E and cancer prevention." *American Journal of Clinical Nutrition*, 53 (1991): 283S-286S.

Knodell, R.G.;Tate, M.A.; Aki, B.F.; and Wilson, J.W. "Vitamin C prophylaxis for post-transfusion hepatitis: Lack of effect in a controlled trial." *American Journal of Clinical Nutrition*, 34 (1981): 20-23.

Kornhauser, A.; Wamer, W.G.; Wei, R.R.; Lambert, L.A.; and Lavu, W. "Timmer antioxidants and cancer prevention in vivo and in vitro." Denver, Co: Second Denver Conference on Nutrition and Cancer, Sept 7-11, 1994.

Lamm, D.L.; Riggs, D.R.; Shriver, J.S.; VanGilder, P.F.; Rach, J.F. and DeHaven, J.I. "Megadose vitamins in bladder cancer: A double blind clinical trial." *The Journal of Urology*, 151 (1994): 21-26.

Lee, I.; Kim, J.H.; Levitt, S.H.; and Song, C.W. "Increases in tumor response by pentoxifyllin alone or in combination with nicotinamide." *International Journal of Radiation Oncology, Biology, Physics*, 322: 425-429.

Lee, I. and Song, C.W. "The oxygenization of murine tumor isografts and human tumor xenografts by nicotinamide." *Radiation Research*, 130 (1992): 65-71.

LeGardeur, B.Y.; Lopez, A.; and Johnson, W.D. "A case-control study of serum vitamins A, E, and C in lung cancer patients." *Nutrition and Cancer*, 14 (1990): 133-140.

Levine, A.M. "The Importance of Hope." *West Journal of Medicine*, 150 (1989): 609.

Levine, M.; Conry-Cantilena, C.; Wang, Y.; Welch, R.W.; Washko, P.W.; Dhariwal, K.R.; Park, J.B.; Lazarev, A.; Graumlich, J.F.; King, J.; and Cantilena, L.R. "Vitamin C pharmacokinetics in healthy volunteers: Evidence for a recommended dietary allowance." *Proceedings of the National Academy of Sciences*, 93 (1995): 3704-3709.

Lewin, S. *Vitamin C: Its molecular biology and medical potential.* New York, NY: Academic Press, 1976.

Lian, S.L.; Hsu, H.Y.; and Lin, S.M. "Serum copper and zinc levels in patients with nasophryngeal carcinoma." *Journal of the Formosan Medical Association*, 88 (1989): 236-239.

Longnecker, M.P.; Martin-Morreno, J.M.; Knekt, P.; Nomura, A.M.; Schober, S.E.; Staheiin, H.B.; Wald, N.J.; Gey, K.F.; and Willett, W.C. "Serum alpha-tocopherol con

centrations in relation to subsequent colorectal cancer: Pooled data from five cohorts." *Journal of the National Cancer Institute*, 84 (1992): 430-435.

MacFarlane, J.K. "Carcinoma of the pancreas: Confessions of a frustrated surgical oncologist." *Annals RCPSC*, 24 (1991): 293-296.

McCracken, R.D. *Niacin and Human Health Disorders*. Fort Collins, CO: Hygea Publishing Co., n.d.

McKeown-Eyysen, G.; Holloway, C.; Jazmaji, V.; Bright-See, E.; Dion, P.; and Bruce, W.R. "A randomized trial of vitamins C and E in the prevention of recurrence of colorectal polyps." *Cancer Research*, 48 (1988): 4701-4705.

Mann, D.M.A. and Yates, P.O. "Possible role of neuromelanin in the pathogenesis of Parkinson's disease." *Mechanism of Ageing and Development*, 21 (1990): 32-38.

Matthews, S.B.; Henderson, A.H.; and Campbell, A.K. "The adrenochrome pathway: The major route for adrenalin catabolism by polymorphonuclear leucocytes." *Journal of Mol Cell Cardiology*, 17 (1985): 339-348.

Moertel, C.G.; Fleming,T.R.; Creagan, E.T.; Rubin, J.; O'Connell, M.J.; and Ames, M.M. "High-dose vitamin C versus placebo in the treatment of patients with advanced cancer who had no prior chemotherapy." *New England Journal of Medicine*, 312 (1985): 137-141.

Moertel, S.G. "Current concepts in cancer: Chemotherapy of gastrointestinal cancer." *New England Journal of Medicine*, 299 (1978): 1049-1052.

Morishige, F. and Murata, A. "Prolongation of survival times in terminal human cancer by administration of supplemental ascorbate." *Journal of International Academy of Preventative Medicine*, 5 (1979): 47-52.

Moss, R. *The Cancer Industry*. New York, NY: Equinox Press, 1992.

Moyers, B. *Healing and The Mind*. New York NY: Doubleday, 1993.

Nakagawa, K.; Miyazaka, M.; Okui, K.; Kato, N.; Moriyama, Y.; and Fujimura, S. "N-methylnicotinamide level in the blood after nicotinamide loading as further evidence for malignant tumor burden." *Japanese Journal of Cancer Research*, 82 (1991): 1277-1283.

Nakatsugawa, S. and Sugahara, T. "Differential action on cancer and normal tissue by adrenochrome monaminoguanidine methanesulfonate and cytochrome C combined with radiotherapy." *International Journal of Radiation Oncology, Biology, Physics*, 29 (1994): 635-638.

Nauts, H.C. "Bacterial products in the treatment of cancer: Past, present and future." *Bacteria and Cancer* (Jeljaszewics, J.; Pulverer, G. and Rostowski, W., eds.). New York, NY: Academic Press, 1982.

Noto, V.; Taper, H.S.; Yi-Hya, J.; Janssens, J.; Bonte, J.; and De Loecker, W. "Effects of sodium ascorbate (vitamin C) and 2-methyl-l4 naphthoquinone (vitamin K3) treatment on human tumor cell growth in vitro. 1. Synergism of combined vitamin C and K3 action." *Cancer*, 63 (1989): 901-906.

Olanow, C.W. "Oxidization reactions in Parkinson's disease." *Neurology*, 40, Supp 3 (1990): 32-38.

Padh, H. "Vitamin C: Newer insights into its biochemical functions." *Nutrition Reviews*, 49 (1991): 65-70.

Palan, P.R.; Mikhail, M.S.; and Romney, S.L. "Plasma levels of antioxidant beta-carotene and alpha tocopherol in uterine cervix dysplasia and cancer." *Nutrition and Cancer*, 15 (1991): 13-20.

Parsons, W.B.; Achor, R.W.P.; Berge, K.G. et al. "Changes in concentration of blood lipid levels following prolonged administration of large doses of nicotinic acid to persons with hypercholesterolemia: preliminary observations." *Proc. Staff. Meet Mayo Clinic*, 31 (1956): 377-390.

Parsons, B.W. *Clinical Alternatives. Coronary Heart Disease. The Dietary Sense and Nonsense. An Evaluation by Scientists.* Ed. G.V.Mann. London, UK: Janus Publishing Co., 1993.

Pauling, L. "Biostatistical analysis of mortality data for cohorts of cancer patients." *Proceedings of the National Academy of Sciences, USA*, 86:3466-3488, 1989.

Pauling, L. "Orthomolecular Psychiatry," *Science*, 160 (1968): 265-271.

Pauling, L. *Vitamin C and the Common Cold.* San Francisco, CA: W.H. Freeman, 1971.

Pauling, L. *How To Live Longer and Feel Better*. New York, NY: W.H.Freeman & Co., 1986.

Pauling, L. Quoted by J. Challen, in *The Nutrition Reporter*, 3, 8, 1992.

Pauling, L. and Herman, Z. "Criteria for the validity of clinical trials of treatments of cohorts of cancer patients based on the Hardin Jones principle." *Proceedings of the National Academy of Sciences*, 86 (1989): 6835-6837.

Pfeiffer, C.C. *Zinc and Other Micro-Nutrients*. New Canaan, CT: Keats Publishing, Inc., 1978.

Prasad, K.N. and Rama, B.N. "Nutrition and cancer." *1984-85 Yearbook of Nutritional Medicine*. J. Bland, ed. New Canaan, CT: Keats Publishing Inc., 1985.

Prasad, K.N. "Vitamins induce cell proliferation, growth inhibition and enhance the effect of tumor therapeutic agents on some cancer cells in culture." Denver, CO: Second Denver Conference on Nutrition and Cancer, Sept 7-11, 1994.

Prasad, K.N. "Cellular basis of using multiple antioxidant vitamins in cancer prevention and treatment." Tampa, FL: Nutrition in Cancer Treatment Symposium, 1995.

Prasad, N.; Santamaria, L.; and Williams, R.M., eds. *Nutrients in Cancer Prevention and Treatment*. New Jersey: Humana Press, 1995: 363-72.

Richards, E. "The politics of therapeutic evaluation: The vitamin C and cancer controversy." *Soc. Stud. of Science*, 18 (1988): 653-701.

Richards, E. *Vitamin C and Cancer - Medicine or Politics?* London, UK: Macmillan Professional and Academic Ltd., 1991.

Rimm, E.B.; Stampfer, M.J.; Ascherio, A.; Giovannucci, E.; Colditz, G.A.; and Willett, W.C. "Vitamin E consumption and the risk of coronary heart disease in men." *New England Journal of Medicine*, 328 (1993): 1450-1456.

Riordan, H.D.; Jackson, J.A.; and Schulz, M. "Case study: High-dose intravenous vitamin C in the treatment of a patient with adenocarcinoma of the kidney." *Journal of Orthomolecular Medicine*, 5 (1990): 5-7.

Rogers, M.A.; Thomas, D.B.; Weiss, N.S.; Vaughan, T.L.; and Nevissi, A.E. "A case control study of oral cancer and prediagnostic concentrations of selenium and zinc in nail tissue." *International Journal of Cancer*, 48 (1991): 182-188.

Rueff, D. "Clinical experience with antioxidant supplementation in oncological treatments. Therapeutic potential of biological antioxidants." Tiburon, CA: Linus Pauling Institute of Science & Medicine, September 29-October 1, 1994.

Sapolsky, R.M. "On Human Nature." *The Sciences*, 34 (1994):10-12.

Schapira, A.H.V.; Cooper, J.M.; Dexter, D.; Clark, J.B.; Jenner, P.; and Marsden, C.D. "Mitochondrial complex I deficiency in Parkinson's disease." *Journal of Neurochemistry*, 54 (1990): 823-827.

Scheulin, M.E.; Schmitt-Graff, A.; and Schmidt, C.G. "Reduction of adriamycin cardiotoxicity by niacin and isocitrate." *Proceedings of the 74th Annual Meeting, American Association for Cancer Research*, 24 (1983): 251.

Schmitt-Graff, A. and Scheulen, M.E. "Prevention of adriamycin cardiotoxicity by niacin, isocitrate or N-acetyl-cysteine in mice." *Path. Res. Pract.*, 181 (1985): 168-174.

Slevin, M.L. "Quality of life: Philosophical question or clinical reality?" *British Medical Journal*, 305 (1992): 466-469.

Smythies, J. "On the function of neuromelanin." *Proceedings of the Royal Society (London)*, B263 (1996): 491-496.

Smythies, J. "Hallucinogenic drugs." *Encyclopedia of Neuroscience*, 1996.

Smythies, J. "The role of ascorbate in brain: Therapeutic implications." *Journal of the Royal Society of Medicine*, 89 (1996): 241.

Smythies, J. "Disturbances of one-carbon metabolism in neuropsychiatric disorders: A review." Submitted to *Biological Psychiatry*, 1996.

Stampfer, M.J.; Hennekens, C.H.; Manson, J.; Colditz, G.A.; Rosner, B.; and Willett, C. "Vitamin E consumption and the risk of coronary disease in women." *New England Journal of Medicine*, 328 (1993): 1444-1449.

Stone, I. *The Healing Factor: Vitamin C against Disease*. New York, NY: Grosset and Dunlap, 1972.

Streffer, C. "The biosynthesis of NAD in the liver of irradiated mice." *Journal of Vitaminology*, 14 (1968): 130-134.

Sugamoto, K.; Kimura, H.; Kawashima, H.; Itojima, T.; Aoyama, T.; and Sugahara, T. "Radioprotective effects of adrenochrome monoaminoguanidine methanesulfonate (AMM) on irradiated C57Bl mice and the survival of GM-CFC, a hemotopoietic progenitor cell." *Journal of Radiation Research*, 29 (1988): 211-219.

Tannock, I. Reported in *The Medical Post*, Oct 18, 1934, page 16, by Louise Gagnon.

Titus, K. "Scientists link niacin and cancer prevention." *The D.O.*, 28 (1987): 93-97.

Toke, G.B. and Dhamne, B.K. "A study of serum copper, serum zinc and Cu/Zn ratio as diagnostic and prognostic index in cases of head, neck and face tumors." *Indian Journal of Pathology and Microbiology*, 33 (1990): 171-174.

Toma, S.; Micheletti, A.; Giacherro, P.; Coialbu, T.; Collechi, P.; Esposito, M.; Rotondi, M.; Albanese, E.; and Cantoni, E. "Selenium therapy in patients with precancerous and malignant oral cavity lesions: Preliminary results." *Cancer Detection and Prevention*, 15 (1991): 491-494.

Trivers, E.R. *Zinc, An Essential Trace Element*. Buena Park, CA: Committee for World Health, 1991.

Vickers, A. "The NIH methodology conference: The methodology debate in the United Kingdom during the past ten years." *Journal of Alternative and Complementary Medicine*, 1 (1995): 167-170.

Wahrendorf, J.; Munoz, N.; Lu, J.B.; Thurnham, D.I.; Crespi, M. and Bosch, F.X. "Blood, retinal and zinc riboflavin status in relation to precancerous lesions of the esophagus: Findings from a vitamin intervention trial in the Peoples Republic of China." *Cancer Research*, 48: 2280-2283.

Werbach, M.R. *Nutritional Influences on Illness: A Sourcebook of Clinical Research*. Tarzana, CA: Third Line Press, 1987.

Williams, R.J. *You Are Extraordinary*. New York, NY: Random House, Inc., 1967.

Williams, R.J. *Nutrition against Disease*. New York, NY: Pitman Pub. Corp., 1971.

Williams, R.J. *Physician's Handbook of Nutritional Science*. Springfield, IL: C.C. Thomas, 1975.

Winn, R.J. and Levin, B. "Chemoprevention of colon cancer. New Perspectives in Large Bowel Cancer." *Hematology/Oncology Clinics of North America*, 3 (1989): 65-75.

Wood, P.J.; Counsell, C.J.; Bremner, J.C.; Horsman, M.R.; and Adams, G.E. "The measurement of radiosensitizer-induced changes in mouse tumor metabolism by 31P magnetic resonance spectroscopy." *International Journal of Radiation Oncology, Biology, Physics*, 20 (1991): 291-294.

Woodward, B. "Zinc, a pharmacologically potent essential nutrient: Focus on immunity." *Canadian Medical Association Journal*, 145: 1469.

Yamashita, H.; Okura, J. and Izumi, K. "Protective effect of adrenochrome monoguanylhydrazone methanesulfonate (S Adchon) on the hematopoietic organ as revealed in irradiated cancer patients." *Journal of Radiation Research*, 12 (1971): 41-50.

Yu. S.; Mai, B.; Xiao, P.; Yu, W.; Wang, Y.; Huang, C.; Chen, W. ; and Xuan, X. "Intervention trial with selenium for the prevention of lung cancer among tin miners in Yunnan, China. A pilot study." *Biological Trace Element Research*, 24 (1990): 105-108.